TH

Andreas Michalsen, MD, PhD, is a professor of clinical complementary medicine at the Charité University Medical Center, Berlin, the largest university hospital in Europe. He is also head of the Department of Internal and Complementary Medicine at Immanuel Hospital, Berlin. Dr. Michalsen is board certified in internal medicine, emergency medicine, and physical medicine and rehabilitation. He has published more than two hundred scientific articles in top medical journals and has collaborated with Stanford University, Harvard University, the University of Southern California, the Mayo Clinic, and many other institutions.

\* \* \*

## Praise for *The Nature Cure*

"Michalsen advocates for and explains the science behind leeching, fasting, meditation, yoga, and vegetarianism. I loved it."     —*New York Magazine*

"Most people don't know that water actually can promote healing in other ways besides quenching our thirst. . . . [Michalsen] discusses how we can use the practice of hydrotherapy in our everyday lives, as well as the importance of using water as a healing tool."     —*MindBodyGreen*

"Full of science and research, [Dr. Michalsen] returns to the earth and shares how we, too, can use the natural world around us to feel better."
—*Read It Forward*

"Integration of conventional medicine and naturopathic medicine makes good sense. Dr. Andreas Michalsen believes, as I do, in the healing power of nature. In this informative book, he demonstrates the safety and efficacy of time-honored methods of optimizing health and treating illness, including dietary adjustment, applications of heat and cold, the use of natural remedies, fasting, and therapies derived from Ayurvedic and Traditional Chinese Medicine. I recommend it to practitioners and patients alike."
—Andrew Weil, MD, author of *Eight Weeks to Optimum Health*
and *Mind over Meds*

"A wonderful resource to guide anyone seeking to improve their health or reverse the suffering from chronic disease."
—Terry Wahls, MD, author of *The Wahls Protocol*

"[Dr. Michalsen] is one of the best doctors of natural medicine I have ever known. His therapies are based on solid scientific and clinical pillars. In the field of therapeutic fasting, his clinic in Berlin is among the most prestigious in the world and is at the forefront of experimentation and implementation of new scientific discoveries on patients with diseases ranging from hypertension and diabetes to cancer and multiple sclerosis. This is a book that brings us toward a new approach to medicine, a book that is not to be missed."  —Valter Longo, PhD, author of *The Longevity Diet*

"Here is a clear and straightforward guide to healing like no other in print. Professor Michalsen is a world expert in natural health approaches, and now he makes his wisdom available to all. A wonderful book that will help anyone who reads it heal."

—Wayne B. Jonas, MD, author of *How Healing Works*

"Essential reading for anyone interested in living a long and healthy life. Filled with compelling research and gripping stories of Dr. Michalsen's own patients, *The Nature Cure* reveals the simple and accessible changes we can make to live well."  —Dr. Qing Li, author of *Forest Bathing*

"Dr. Andreas Michalsen has impeccable medical credentials and has been curing thousands upon thousands of patients for more than thirty years. With *The Nature Cure*, we now all have access to his wisdom on preventing and treating diseases. This scientifically-based and accessible book will help to transform lives as it contains a multitude of actionable recommendations to reverse and prevent multiple diseases."

—Lorenzo Cohen, PhD, professor and director of the Integrative
Medicine Program at MD Anderson Cancer Center and
coauthor of *Anticancer Living*

"A professor of clinical complementary medicine at the Charité University Medical Center Berlin explores the power and potential of natural medicine."  —*Publishers Weekly*

"Sprinkled with case studies throughout, the book provides inspiration and more evidence that natural therapies can and do heal. . . . DIY health readers and fans of natural medicine will find this title scientifically validating and filled with new information."  —*Library Journal*

# The

# NATURE

# CURE

*A Doctor's Guide to the*
*Science of Natural Medicine*

ANDREAS MICHALSEN, MD, PhD

*with* PETRA THORBRIETZ

life

PENGUIN BOOKS
An imprint of Penguin Random House LLC
penguinrandomhouse.com

First published in the United States of America by Viking,
an imprint of Penguin Random House LLC, 2019
Published in Penguin Books 2020

This work was originally published in German as *Heilen mit der Kraft der Natur* by
Insel Verlag Berlin. This Penguin edition is published by arrangement with Insel Verlag Berlin.

This work was translated by Laura Wagner.
The German-language edition was edited by Friedrich-Karl Sandmann.

Illustrations by Tom Menzel, tigercolor: pp. 39, 56, 100, 208.
All other illustrations: Sofarobotnik, Augsburg & Munich.

ISBN 9780525561293 (paperback)

THE LIBRARY OF CONGRESS HAS CATALOGED THE HARDCOVER EDITION AS FOLLOWS:
Title: The nature cure: a doctor's guide to the science of natural medicine /
Andreas Michalsen, MD with Petra Thorbrietz.
Other titles: Heilen mit der Kraft der Natur. English
Description: New York: Viking, 2019. |
Identifiers: LCCN 2019011636 (print) | LCCN 2019018339 (ebook) |
ISBN 9780525561286 (ebook) | ISBN 9780525561279 (hardcover)
Subjects: LCSH: Naturopathy. | Alternative medicine. | BISAC: Health &
Fitness / Naturopathy. | Medical / Holistic Medicine. | Medical /
Alternative Medicine.
Classification: LCC RZ433 (ebook) | LCC RZ433 .M5313 2019 (print) |
DDC 615.5/35—dc23
LC record available at https://lccn.loc.gov/2019011636

Printed in the United States of America

Set in Minion Pro
Designed by Gretchen Achilles

# Contents

# Foreword

*By Valter Longo, PhD*

For hundreds of years health has been managed, on one hand, by official medicine, based on the teachings of medical schools at the most important universities, on the results of clinical studies, and on the decisions of government agencies. On the other hand, health has also been managed by complementary medicine—sometimes based on ancient traditions, sometimes of dubious origin. In *The Nature Cure*, Dr. Andreas Michalsen combines the teachings of official medicine and science-based complementary medicine to help readers live healthier while minimizing the need for medication. Dr. Michalsen starts with the story of his personal journey to naturopathic medicine and then comes to discuss a variety of naturopathic therapies ranging from the use of leeches, hydrotherapy, yoga, exercise, diet and fasting, and how they can prevent and even cure major diseases. Dr. Michalsen, head of the naturopathy department at the Immanuel Hospital and Charité Medical University in Berlin, is one of the best doctors of natural medicine I have ever known. His therapies are based on solid scientific and clinical pillars. In the field of therapeutic fasting, his clinic

in Berlin is among the most prestigious in the world and is at the forefront of experimentation and implementation of new scientific discoveries on patients with diseases ranging from hypertension, diabetes,
and cancer to multiple sclerosis. This is a book that brings us toward a
new approach to medicine, a book that is not to be missed.

# Introduction

Fasting, yoga, Ayurveda, herbal medicine, meditation, mindfulness, a vegetarian diet—the subjects of naturopathy are more topical than ever before. But it's difficult to find scientifically-founded guidance on naturopathy. Some things that have long been recommended in the world of natural medicine should be questioned critically. On the other hand, effective methods of naturopathy are often too quickly dismissed by conventional physicians. Yet it's become increasingly clear that many people are interested in exploring naturopathy and integrative medicine. It is high time, then, for an evaluation that takes experience, practice, and research into consideration in equal measure.

Medicine needs naturopathy—now more urgently than ever before. An increasing number of chronic diseases is becoming widespread, and conventional medicine's method of treating these illnesses in the same highly technologized manner as emergency cases—with surgeries, interventions, and new medications—leads to more and more side effects and unaffordable costs.

The traditional treatment methods of naturopathy have kept people alive throughout the centuries and have addressed various illnesses with astonishing efficacy—even though the methods were based solely on practical experience. Then modern medicine came along with its scientific approach and its extraordinary possibilities for diagnosis and therapy, and a lot of ancient knowledge was left by the wayside because it was considered outdated or even wrong.

Yet today, the latest research methods of modern biology and medicine show that naturopathy is not a thing of the past, but highly relevant. In the crisis of medicine we're now facing—with its increasing costs and rising proportion of chronic illness—naturopathy offers solutions, showing us new ways of preventing and treating diseases. The central focus is not on the illness, but on the individual.

As professor of Clinical Naturopathy at the Charité Berlin, the largest university hospital in Europe, with about three thousand inpatient beds and more than twelve thousand health professionals and scientists working there, I hope to share the enormous potential of naturopathy with the public and to close the gaps that continually seem to open between "high-tech" medicine and practical knowledge. At the Charité, our focus is not on setting divisions between different ways of medical practice, but on integration and combination—on a scientific basis. Employing this concept, we treat thousands of patients to great success every year.

## MY JOURNEY TO NATUROPATHY

I was born in a small village in the southern part of Germany, on the border of Austria and Switzerland, near the Alps. My father and grandfather were both MDs who specialized in internal medicine. As a child, listening to my father talk about his workday at the dinner table, I realized that there was something special about his medical practice. Following in the tradition of my grandfather, my father treated his patients not only with conventional medication and surgery, but also with naturopathic and integrative medicine. He often advised lifestyle and diet changes for his patients, such as fasting or reducing stress. He didn't just prescribe conventional drugs, but also herbs and supplements. Growing up I was accustomed to seeing his patients stop by our home to express their gratitude and sometimes to drop off a present—usually something nice to eat. On the other hand, I also grew up hearing my father talk about the suspicion with which his colleagues regarded his approach to medicine.

My two siblings and I grew up in a loving home, surrounded by the principles of naturopathy. Our home had hot tubs and a Finnish sauna. My father would take cold baths in the swimming pool in our garden— even during the freezing German winters. We were encouraged to eat vegetables, fruit, and nuts. To drink herbal tea when suffering from a cold. So naturally, this felt like the norm to me—the way medicine should be.

After graduating from high school I decided to study economics and philosophy. Trying to understand the grand scheme of things has never ceased to fascinate me. But unlike other disciplines, medicine seems to be something that puts theory into practice directly, entirely hands-on. And like many young people, I wanted to find a calling that would allow me to help others. Or maybe it was just the family tradition that had me firmly in its grasp. In any case, I kept finding myself in biology lectures and realized that I felt much more comfortable there. So, it was to be medicine, after all.

Back in the eighties, when I was studying, the worldview of scientists was extremely mechanistic. For example, in one of the weekly sessions that were part of my training as an internist, I remember introducing a study exploring how psychological stress could cause a heart attack. As a result, I was ridiculed. "How do you imagine that would happen, Michalsen?" I was asked with pointed derision. "Like, would anger spontaneously create a blood clot?" Yet since then, countless studies have proven that anger and fear actually do constrict the arteries, which can cause blood coagulation and the dangerous blood clots that form the basis of a heart attack.

When I was training to be a doctor, eminence-based medicine was in the process of transforming into evidence-based medicine. Just before, the "demigod" doctor, the eminence, was able to do whatever he thought was right. But suddenly, he was required to prove that his therapies were effective by conducting studies and through properly and systematically documented clinical practice. Evidence-based medicine introduced more rationality into medical practice. But it also began to ignore very simple knowledge and wisdom that wasn't supported by existing studies. Knowledge such as the fact that people fall asleep better when their feet are warm rather than cold. Later it also became clear that research is conducted mainly where there is a return on investment—patentable drugs, in other words. There is little money to be earned from hot footbaths, and it's accordingly difficult to obtain research funding for it.

My superior at the time, Walter Thimme, MD, however, was always open to new findings. He was a very experienced and science-oriented professor, who turned each patient's course of treatment into an exam during rounds. In addition, he was the editor of the pharma-critical magazine Der Arzneimittelbrief, and it was he who taught me that chronically ill patients take far too many drugs and that it's always obligatory to examine what benefit each and every pill actually has for the patient. We had very constructive arguments and he would say, "Why don't you write an article about . . . ." That way, I learned to describe the effect of medicinal plants or the importance of nutrition. On the occasion of his retirement in 2001, he asked me to give a grand round lecture about complementary medicine in cardiology. Those were very positive experiences I had in dialogue with conventional medicine.

No one in my classes shared my background in naturopathy, but there was a study group where we learned about the work of Viktor von Weizsäcker. He advocated an anthropologic-biographical approach to anamnesis—he was concerned with understanding a person's entire history when it came to their medical treatment. This study group was a colorful mixture of aspiring internists, neurologists, and psychiatrists. I still keep in touch with some of them today. All of them are committed to seeing patients in their entirety.

I have always maintained the idea that traditional knowledge and modern medicine don't have to be mutually exclusive. Ideally, they complement each other. The internistic-cardiologic ward of the Humboldt Hospital in Berlin where I trained was huge—ambulances, 120 beds, an intensive care unit—and fascinating, holding all the possibilities medicine had to offer. Our professor had high scientific standards; every week we had to read and discuss the newest relevant articles from the *New England Journal of Medicine*. I thought this scientific aspiration was wonderful. What was practiced in our department was very ambitious conventional medicine, but with a focus on reducing medical intervention—not everyone taking ASS blood thinners, for example, also received a stomachic. And not everyone presenting with chest pains was summoned to the cardiac catheterization lab immediately. Instead, we examined everything in an individual, subjective way.

Unfortunately, cardiology has strayed far from these standards. Because hospitals make money from cardiac catheters, for example, doctors in Germany are quick to insert them—624 times a year per

100,000 citizens. In other OECD member countries this happens only 177 times on average. Is it possible that we are better cared for in Germany than in other comparable countries? Not in this regard. The statistics also show that on average, life expectancy doesn't necessarily rise after a catheter procedure. For acute heart attacks, widening a coronary vessel can save lives—but not if, as it so often happens, it is carried out as a preventative measure. Why do doctors perform a procedure that suggests to patients that their blood vessels can be repaired like ordinary pipes and that they don't have to change anything about their lifestyle? The money insurance companies spend on it would be of much better use elsewhere.

As a young doctor on the cardiologic intensive care unit and in the cardiac catheter lab I began to ask questions like: "What therapeutic consequences does this treatment have for the patient?" This is not an obvious question, because specialized high-performance medicine primarily focuses on the alleviation of acute symptoms. Whether or not a person benefits from a treatment in the long run is not a major concern.

I learned a lot in the "cleanroom," where patients spent about ten to fifteen minutes after their heart catheterization. It was common practice for the doctor carrying out the catheterization to compress the artery in the groin during those ten to fifteen minutes after the tube was removed so that there wouldn't be any bleeding later on. The patients were happy to have come out of the procedure unscathed and glad to have someone to talk to. I often asked patients what they thought had caused their heart problems—a sort of subjective disease evaluation. Every person had a reason to share: "I was under a lot of stress," "I've been unemployed for a while," "It runs in the family," and so on. Even though evaluations like these are often only partially accurate, they still offer crucial details that would never have been mentioned in a normal consult during which the patient is primarily required to listen.

By this time, I had spent eight years mastering the tools of modern cardiology, such as performing heart catheterizations and implanting pacemakers. I had become a certified specialist in internal and cardio-vascular medicine as well as in emergency and critical care medicine, and I'd published scientific works on heart failure.

But during this period I came to realize that although I had these impressive technical treatments at my disposal, I wasn't addressing the real cause of the underlying diseases I was treating. A coronary stent is a great help to a patient with a myocardial infarction. But it doesn't treat the underlying cause of this disease—atherosclerosis. We advised our patients to stop smoking, to change their diets, to exercise, but advocating for lifestyle changes was not the focus of how we prac-ticed medicine.

It was then that I decided to engage in clinical research in nutri-tional medicine, traditional and herbal medicine, lifestyle-based med-icine, and mind-body medicine. I contacted the head of the clinical department of integrative and naturopathic medicine at the Charité University Hospital in Berlin. Here I had my first experiences with clin-ical naturopathy—with fasting, hydrotherapy, acupuncture, and leech therapy.

In 1999, I was appointed deputy director of the first large special-ized hospital for naturopathy and complementary medicine in Bad Elster, Germany. Then in 2001, I moved to the University Hospital in Essen, Germany, where I was appointed deputy director and head of clinical inpatient care in the newly founded department for naturo-pathic and integrative medicine. There I finished my PhD in 2006 and received further certifications in nutritional medicine, physical medi-cine, and rehabilitation.

In 2009, I became head of the Department for Naturopathy at the Immanuel Hospital in Berlin and was called to the endowed professorship for Clinical Naturopathy at the Charité University Hospital, Berlin, the largest university hospital in Europe. We treat more than eight thousand patients a year with naturopathic and integrative medicine across all diseases, but mainly internal diseases. It is the largest academic department of its kind in Europe and America. In fact, more than half of the German Nobel Prize winners in medicine and physiology have come from the Charité.

## WHAT IS NATUROPATHY?

I believe that every single one of us can benefit from incorporating the principles of naturopathy into our lives. But what is naturopathy? For me, naturopathy is the foundation of medicine, particularly in treating chronic illnesses. Naturopathy uses natural elements in treatment, such as diet, fasting, exercise, massage, stress management, sunlight, herbs, and water. All of these things are "natural," so to speak. The principle is always to apply natural support and stimulation to the mind and body, with the aim of enhancing self-healing.

These concepts of natural medicine can be found in different cultures around the world from Europe to America to India to China to Japan. The principles remain the same—they always revolve around the use of natural factors. I do want to say here that other frequently used alternative methods, homeopathy for example, are not naturopathy. This is important to underline in scientific discussions.

I'm continuously surprised by the negativity or controversy surrounding naturopathy. A common misunderstanding is that naturopathy may advise patients to avoid conventional treatment. This is not the purpose of true naturopathy. Naturopathy aims to support or complement conventional medicine—it's the best of both worlds!

In Germany, this is made clear by regulation, as all naturopathic doctors are MDs and have to have a certified specialization in a field of conventional medicine of the German medical association.

Of course it might be possible that the use of naturopathy results in a reduced need for medication. For example, a patient who switches to a plant-based diet might experience a normalization in blood pressure, resulting in a decreased need for medication. This does not put naturopathy at odds with conventional medicine—it's simply a sign of supported self-healing. Similarly, an herbal treatment may result in a reduced need for painkillers, which will help a patient avoid potential serious side effects such as renal failure or gastrointestinal bleeding. These are positive consequences of naturopathy and integrative medicine, and do not mean that naturopathic medicine is opposed to conventional medicine. It's pure synergy.

This combination of conventional and science-based naturopathic medicine is also how more and more patients want to be treated. Over the past several years I've witnessed an increasing demand for naturopathic and integrative medicine. About 60,000 of the 300,000 MDs in Germany already practice some kind of naturopathic and integrative medicine. Accordingly, naturopathy is taught and practiced in the best university hospitals and medical schools in Germany, as the Charité Medical University in Berlin.

I believe that the biggest challenge for twenty-first-century medicine will be the increasing life expectancy in the developed world. If we do not succeed in staying healthy for longer, our increased lifespan will only result in more years of living with disease. Who wants that?

Natural healing, with its complex biological approach, seems to be the right answer for the increasing number of chronic diseases that are the result of stress, an unhealthy diet, and a sedentary and nature-deprived lifestyle. The fact that nature and humans have lived for hundreds of thousands of years in close interdependence explains why natural methods are so powerful in lifestyle-related diseases. As a doctor, medical director, and researcher, I have seen tens of thousands of patients become cured, or at least much improved, through the use of natural integrative therapies such as leech therapy, cupping, acupuncture, Ayurveda, fasting or a plant-based diet, forest bathing, hydrotherapy, yoga, meditation, and tai chi.

The healing power of nature is amazing. Science-based naturopathy can help us live longer and stay healthy as we age. Up to 80 percent of chronic diseases can be prevented or treated by naturopathy and lifestyle methods. Hypertension, diabetes, inflammatory and immune diseases, depression, and many age-related diseases *can* be avoided.

During my years in medical residency the stress of life had a grip on me. Due to the intense workload, I was eating poorly and grappling with high stress levels. As my cholesterol and blood pressure increased, I thought of my grandfather and father and their approach to health. I switched to a plant-based diet and started to meditate and practice yoga, and experienced the profound effects of these methods. Soon my blood tests and blood pressure normalized.

Integrative medicine is a truly global medicine, a "one world" medicine. We have modern fasting techniques from German and American doctors, as well as traditional religious fasting practices in Christianity, Hinduism, Judaism, Islam, and Buddhism. There are the very healthy "blue zones"—where people typically live longer than average—found throughout the world. Leech therapy was practiced in ancient Greece and Rome, as well as in China, India, and in the Amazon. The same is true of cupping. If we look at herbs, they are recommended in a similar way all over the world, from present-day China to ancient monks from Germany. With this book, I'd like to share all the knowledge of science-based naturopathy. My interest in naturopathy has changed my life, and my hope is that this book might motivate you to try naturopathic medicine yourself.

# The
# NATURE
# CURE

# CHAPTER ONE

# The Basic Principles of Naturopathy

### Boosting Self-Healing Powers Through Stimulus and Response

The basic principle of naturopathy—and of all traditional therapies—is the interplay of stimulus and reaction.

For example, let's say you are suffering from a cold. Your doctor is worried that a bacterial pneumonia could attach to the viral infection you already have, so he prescribes an antibiotic as well as an antipyretic. It's his intention to kill the pathogens and to relieve your fever. Maybe you'll also receive a mucolytic—to thin mucus—and zinc or vitamin C to strengthen your immune system.

What approach would naturopathy take?

You would receive a cold, damp chest compress, wound tightly around your body. You would then be wrapped in layers of blankets. This treatment will cool your feverish body down to the point where you might start to shiver, but shortly afterward you'll feel nice and warm, because your body's regulatory systems will have started to fight the cold impulse intensively—and not only locally, i.e., on the surface of the skin, but also on a cellular level. If your temperature continues to rise, leg compresses can be used to counteract the fever.

To induce sweating, you'll be given linden blossom and elderberry tea to drink.

## STIMULATING THE HUMAN BODY

Many stimuli operate in an "unspecific" manner—meaning one particular stimulus can elicit a variety of different reactions in different people based on their individual nerve reflexes and hormone levels. That reactions can differ so greatly on an individual basis—depending on a person's physical constitution and the intensity and frequency of the stimulus—leads some conventional practitioners of medicine to believe that naturopathic treatments don't work. But they're misjudging the principle: While conventional medicine eliminates disease from the outside and often attains quick (but short-lived) successes in doing so, naturopathy works by teasing out our self-healing powers. It aims at stimulating the human body so that we regain our health on our own.

This requires patience. Through deliberately placed and well-dosed stimuli, the body is given a wake-up call to heal. To continue our example from earlier, a patient undergoing a naturopathic treatment for his cold would have to endure his fever (within reason). By doing so he gives his immune system the chance to fight the pathogens itself. He might drink linden blossom tea, which induces sweating. And instead of taking vitamins and antibiotics, which wouldn't help against a virus anyway, he might have a slow-cooked vegetable soup and drink a ginger-turmeric smoothie. Ginger and turmeric contain the best micronutrients in their natural state, which is why they can be more effective than pills.[1, 2]

It's important to place the right stimuli at the right intensity. For a healthy child, fever is important training for the immune system. For an elderly person suffering from a heart condition, fever can be dangerous. The relationship between dosage and effect has become a topic of current international research under the term *hormesis* (from the Greek, meaning "stimulus" or "impulse"). In the sixteenth century, Paracelsus, one of the first pharmacologists of the modern era, realized that a small dose of a poisonous substance can have a positive effect— because the body is introduced to the negative stimulus (noxa) and develops defense mechanisms against it. This same principle is also present in radioactivity, where it's been observed that a low amount of radiation can actually have a positive effect within the body.[3]

However, because there currently just isn't enough data on the exact relationship between dosage and effect of unspecific stimuli, measuring an individual's response is critically important in naturopathy. The most crucial questions about a naturopathic therapy are these types of questions: Did you react well to the broth or the juice cocktail—could you digest it without any problems? Or are your feet getting warm quickly when you're wearing a compress? If the answer is no in both cases, either the dosage or the therapy is not right for you—regardless of whether this dosage or therapy worked on another person in similar circumstances.

## IDENTIFYING THE PATIENT'S PHYSICAL CONSTITUTION

In naturopathy, deciding what stimulus to use depends less on the illness and more on the individual person and her physical constitution. A person's physique, psyche, and bodily regulation are interrelated in a way that can cause certain symptoms and diseases. Though it's sometimes possible to predict what symptoms or diseases a patient might have based on her constitution, such typifying is helpful mainly only as a point of reference. Most people do not fall neatly into categories. Not every obese person with a round belly (the "endomorph") has type 2 diabetes, just as not every overly thin person with pale skin suffers from depression.

So, I would never prescribe a powerful hyperthermic treatment (such as infrared hyperthermia) to someone who generally doesn't like heat, even if the person in question suffers from fibromyalgia, which is often soothed by such a treatment.[4] By the same token, staying in a cold chamber—two to three minutes at negative 166 degrees Fahrenheit—is not helpful to patients with rheumatism, who constantly feel cold despite their propensity to inflammation.

## THE RIGHT DOSAGE: USING THE SUN AS AN EXAMPLE

Over the course of evolution, two things were extremely important for human survival: sunlight and temperature. We can still observe how dependent we are on these two kinds of stimuli as soon as the days grow darker and the nights grow colder. During the winter, many people find themselves getting tired easily. There is even seasonal depression that manifests itself in the winter months, which can be immediately relieved through exposure to bright light.[5]

The sun is an excellent example of hormesis—the biological phenomenon we discussed earlier—in which a small dose of a stimulus is beneficial, but a larger dose of the same stimulus is harmful. A couple decades ago, dermatologists realized that the risk for certain kinds of skin cancer, especially for basal cell carcinoma, is increased by the sun's ultraviolet light—as is the risk for melanoma. We know that it's not sunbathing in and of itself that causes cancer, but the number of sunburns suffered, though it's still a mystery why melanoma often appears on parts of the body that are hardly ever exposed to the sun, like the soles of the feet.[6] New theories suggest that our immune system constantly fights melanoma cancer cells all over the body, but a sunburn keeps our immune system so busy that cancer cannot be sufficiently warded off in another part of the body.[7]

The popularity of tanning salons is diminishing because of the undisputed fact that ultraviolet light facilitates skin aging and wrinkles and increases the risk of cancer. But scientific studies also indicate that sunlight makes us happier and increases our well-being.[8] Tanning on UV-A sunbeds is enough to achieve this.[9] UV-B sunbeds are even better, but they cannot be found in normal tanning salons. Decades ago, sunbathing was prescribed for patients with tuberculosis or for people who worked underground. Since 1980, it's been known that sunlight has a positive effect even in cases of severe illness: In his research, Cedric Garland, epidemiologist at the University of California San Diego, found that in areas where the sun shines often, many types of cancer occur far less frequently.[10]

Many autoimmune diseases, such as multiple sclerosis and rheumatoid arthritis, but also heart attacks, some types of cancer, and diabetes, occur more frequently in areas that lie farther north and at a greater distance from the equator.[11] Taking other factors into account, such as a difference in nutrition or social systems, there remains hardly any doubt that the migration of prehistoric humans to the north roughly forty thousand years ago came at the price of an increase in chronic diseases.

Sunlight is also important because it contributes to the creation of a vitamin in our skin that fulfills many essential functions: vitamin D. Vitamin D regulates our bone metabolism, prevents osteoporosis, and also helps protect us from cardiovascular diseases, cancer, depression, and autoimmune diseases. According to recent surveys, 26 percent of the general population in the United States have low levels of vitamin D.[12] A vitamin D deficiency is problematic in old age since the body's ability to synthesize it decreases. This is especially critical because cancer and many other chronic illnesses occur more often in this stage of life. Muscular strength—a key factor for mobility—also diminishes with age. Naturopathy's insistence that it is important to go outside has a purpose. Being outdoors is how we soak up the power of the sun, even when the sky is overcast. Nutrition covers only about 5 percent of our need for vitamin D.[13, 14] You simply cannot substitute time spent in sunlight with a special diet.

The sun presents us with a classic dilemma regarding dosage of stimuli. On the one hand, too much sun exposure can cause skin aging and even skin cancer. On the other hand, we need sunlight for our well-being and the prevention of chronic diseases and cancer. We have to find a compromise.

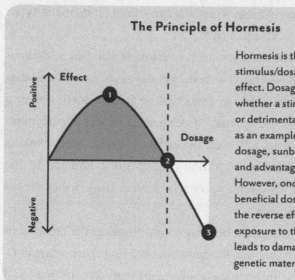

### The Principle of Hormesis

Hormesis is the interplay of stimulus/dosage and reaction/effect. Dosage determines whether a stimulus is beneficial or detrimental. Using sunlight as an example: Up to a certain dosage, sunbathing is beneficial and advantageous to our health. However, once the peak of the beneficial dose is exceeded (1), the reverse effect sets in (2), and exposure to the sun's radiation leads to damage to skin and genetic material (3).

## LIVING IN HARMONY WITH NATURE

Naturopathy means living in accordance with nature, rather than against it. Recent studies show that it's not a simple romantic longing that lies behind this recommendation, but physical fact. There is an evolutionarily shaped connection between our bodies and the natural world. For example, our bodies' biorhythms change according to the seasons. In a 2014 study, researchers from Cambridge and Munich were able to demonstrate that our genetic activity changes depending on the season. About a quarter of our genes react to climate and geographic features; this can even be observed in infants.[15] Nature has provided our bodies with the flexibility to adapt to our environment— an important factor in the success of human evolution.

There exists a sensitive balance between stress factors and protective reactions: Our bodies have a higher propensity for inflammation during winter—probably in order to fight the heightened number of germs and bacteria at that time of year. But as a result, the risk of heart attacks, rheumatism, and diabetes also rises. The control gene ARNTL is tasked with staving off inflammation in the body, but it refrains from doing so in winter to better fight cold and infections. It also regulates body temperature and sleep behavior. This explains why we like to sleep in as the days grow shorter and are generally more lethargic in winter than we are in summer.[16] All in all, there's always a balance that our immune system has to maintain in the midst of seasonal influences.

If we now think about temperature—to what point is the cold a positive stimulus and when does it become unhealthy? Can we train our bodies to be less sensitive to cold temperatures? The answer is yes and no. Compared to the possibility of training a muscle, our ability to adapt to heat and cold is rather low. This is particularly noticeable in the summer, because our bodies struggle to deal with high temperatures over prolonged periods of time. One way our bodies deal with heat is through sweating. Since sweat evaporates quickly, we can lose about 3.5 liters of liquid an hour. If we find ourselves in a hot environment for several weeks, our ability to sweat can double.[17] There's an additional advantage to sweating, in that it makes us lose salt. For those who have a diet high in salt, which is probably most of us, sweating creates a neat offset and enables us to enjoy a buttered pretzel every now and again. People who barely sweat should use the salt shaker with restraint.

To the cold, on the other hand, our bodies react by shivering. First, muscles in minuscule skin vessels contract: This reduces the blood flow to the surface, minimizing the loss of heat. (We sometimes notice this happening when our hands or feet are particularly cold.) The internal organs, however, receive increased blood supply, whereby the body's core temperature is held consistently. If this is still not enough for the body to resist the cold, the muscles underneath the skin tense up. This tension creates warmth. From a certain degree of tension onward the muscles also begin to shiver. Through this forceful contraction, the body tries to turn on a sort of central heating system. Finally, our bodies react to temperature stimuli by changing the isolation layer: In a Japanese study, women were asked to wear either short or long skirts during winter. Using magnetic resonance imaging, researchers were able to show that the women who wore short skirts and presumably had been colder had more fat on their legs by the end of the winter.[18]

## THE POWER OF COLD AND WARM STIMULI

To a certain degree, we can influence our own heat production and train ourselves to be less susceptible to the cold. Sebastian Kneipp, one of the forefathers of modern naturopathy, advised his patients not to stay in heated rooms all the time, but rather to expose themselves to comparatively cool temperatures of 64 to 66 degrees. Cold stimuli— such as Scotch hose therapy using cold water (see page 56), treading in cold water or snow, and cold baths after a sauna—can send signals to the body to make it increase its own heat production. As children, many of us experienced the sensation of burning hands when we returned to our warm homes after a snowball fight. In that scenario, when we suddenly move from a cold to a warm environment, our body dilates or opens its vessels so that blood can flow more easily. This fluctuation between vasoconstriction (in the cold) and vasodilation (in the warmth) is one of the basic principles of Kneipp therapies.

In my hometown of Berlin there are hardened ice bathers who take short baths in frozen lakes even in winter—when the water temperature is 40 degrees. Though this is quite impressive, it is important not to expose the body to any shock. We must train the body's adaptability gradually and systematically by going into cold water for a very short time initially and slowly prolonging the bath.

At the beginning of any cold therapy there needs to be a stable feeling of warmth. For example, feet should be warm before the legs receive a cold Scotch hose treatment. At the Immanuel Hospital in Berlin, we sometimes send patients to a cold chamber where the temperature is negative 166 degrees. But before entering the coldest chamber, patients are sent through two slightly warmer chambers to allow their bodies to adjust to the minimum temperature. They wear nothing but hats, gloves, and warm socks. In the end, they stand in this extreme cold for a maximum of three minutes. The effects are impressive. Pain disappears and inflammations are dulled for hours, even days.

Another phenomenon of bodily regulation was uncovered in recent years: brown fat. Brown fat is special fat tissue that humans—as well as all newborn mammals (with the exception of pigs)—possess. Brown fat cells are packed with mitochondria, which produce energy, and which give the cells their brownish color and create warmth through oxidation. Brown fat protects newborns from becoming hypothermic and helps animals raise their temperatures when emerging from hibernation.

Though it was once believed that adults hardly possess any brown fat, studies conducted by the biologist Wouter van Marken Lichtenbelt in Maastricht show that adults are able to store more brown fat if they are exposed to cool temperatures for prolonged periods of time.[19] This happens at a temperature of 60 degrees. Brown fat facilitates sugar regulation and reduces the risk of getting diabetes. It is healthy, in other words, to stay in cool, slightly uncomfortable, rooms for hours on end. Your body will get used to the low temperatures after a couple of days. People who tend to feel cold quickly should still seek out the cold in order to train their system with short provocations.

Sebastian Kneipp's recommendation to sleep with open windows was affirmed by a study conducted by the National Institute of Diabetes and Digestive and Kidney Diseases: At night, one group slept in a cool room with a maximum temperature of 66 degrees. The other group slept in a room with temperatures higher than 75 degrees. After one month, the group that slept in cool temperatures showed more brown fat in their bodies, and their sugar and fat metabolisms were improved.[20] So, remember: Open windows in the bedroom!

## ON THE DIGESTIVE FIRE AND THE WARMTH OF LIFE

The understanding of energies is more sophisticated both in Ayurveda—the traditional Indian medicine—and in Traditional Chinese Medicine (TCM) than it is in European naturopathy. In both systems, "life warmth" plays a preeminent role. In Ayurvedic medicine, everything revolves around agni, the digestive fire, while in Chinese naturopathy kidney warmth is central. According to both traditions, we should tend to our inner warmth and stoke the digestive fire when temperatures outside are down. The easiest way to do this is by eating certain foods and drinking hot water or tea, especially with the addition of warming spices. It is no coincidence that it is these spices that are used in our holiday cookies, i.e., during the cold season: cloves, cinnamon, ginger, or cardamom. It's good to drink ginger tea or eat heavily seasoned soups (with mustard seeds or chili) on chilly days. Similarly, chicken soup is particularly satisfying on cold days not because of the chicken, but because of the spices it contains, like ginger, onion, or garlic.

Both Ayurveda and Traditional Chinese Medicine divide food-stuffs into "cool" and "warm" categories—a simple but generally help-ful guide for decisions. Cucumber and melon, for example, are cooling, while most savory or hot spices, wine, or honey are warming. In the past, seasonally available foodstuffs corresponded to the seasons. Today, however, one can eat strawberries or watermelon on an icy, freezing day in January. But instinctively, most people choose not to do so. Watermelon for dessert on Christmas Eve? Probably not.

Alcohol is not a remedy for the cold. A beverage high in alcohol con-tent may warm you up in the short run and convey a feeling of warmth in your belly. But since it also facilitates heat emission, you actually end up losing heat faster. So after a snowball fight or an ice bath, it's better to opt for a nonalcoholic herb-and-spice tea rather than a brandy.

Our body's ability to generate heat in response to a cold stimulus isn't always "turned on"—a lack of exercise, fatigue, stress, or a poor diet can contribute to this. In these cases, naturopathy has a stronger method at the ready: hyperthermic baths (also known as Schlenz baths, after the Austrian naturopath Maria Schlenz). These baths can be taken in your bathtub at home: You start with a water temperature of 98.6 degrees (equal to body temperature) and keep running the wa-ter hotter and hotter, until the limit of your comfort is reached. The bath takes twenty to thirty minutes.

Being in a sauna can also work, but since water is a better conduc-tor of heat than air, a hyperthermic bath gets more intense results. You can also utilize the warmth-inducing effect of spices. Adding pow-dered ginger to the bath will allow you to feel the pleasant effect of the heat even more. After taking a hyperthermic bath, you should not seek to cool down immediately as you would after going into a sauna. Instead, you should allow the heat to release fully.

Body temperature can most effectively be heightened by water-filtered infrared radiation of the whole body. This type of treatment involves hyperthermia induced by infrared light. In order not to increase the skin temperature too much, which would be uncomfortable or even painful, the infrared light is water-filtered. This leads to a warming effect two to five centimeters under the skin, hence in the deeper tissue, making this treatment very helpful for treating pain like the kind of pain that occurs as a result of fibromyalgia. A single water-filtered infrared radiation treatment can also notably improve the mood of depressed patients—current research demonstrates that the effect lasts for over two weeks.[21] The exact cause of this astonishing effect is not quite clear, though we can note that people with depression are often cold and sweat less. Hyperthermia activates mitochondria, which are functionally impaired in the brains of people suffering from depression. Interestingly, mitochondria are also thought to be significantly responsible for aging processes, and so the lower percentage of inflammatory and cardiovascular age-related illnesses in the warm, southern parts of the world could be related to that.

---

**PATIENT HISTORY**

## Fibromyalgia
*Persevering Through Pain Is Not the Answer*

The lively woman is in her early sixties. Her gray hair—styled into a short bob—is dyed pink. She's one to keep her chin up, even though she's faced many challenges over the course of her life. During the German Democratic Republic (GDR), or Communist

East Germany, she was sent to prison for political reasons. Years later, in Western Germany, she worked as a waitress and set up her own ice cream parlor. But at some point she found she was no longer able to walk more than fifty meters or climb a flight of stairs. Her arms refused to work. She could hardly carry anything, let alone heavy serving trays. She lost her ice cream parlor and found herself a victim of old-age poverty. Eventually, she was diagnosed with fibromyalgia.

We still don't understand what causes the mysterious pains that occur all over the body with fibromyalgia. Back in the day, the disease was called "soft-tissue rheumatism," but since no physical markers can be detected with blood tests, there are still many doctors who believe psychological problems are the actual cause. Patients with fibromyalgia often feel misunderstood and can develop depression.

Today we know that fibromyalgia is most likely a result of a complex interplay of dysfunctional pain processing in the nerve cells, an overload due to stress and trauma, as well as subtle disturbances of hormone regulation. There is no conventional medical treatment with drugs, except for certain antidepressants that lower pain sensitivity but that are also fraught with side effects.

In naturopathy, there have been some successful treatment options for fibromyalgia. One option is cold or warm therapy, depending on which is more pleasant for the patient. Cold or warm therapy blocks the transmission of pain signals. Another option is meditative exercises like yoga or tai chi. Yet another option is fasting, which intervenes in the body's neurotransmitter environment that plays an important role in the transmission of pain.

The patient started doing tai chi and qigong. These exercises have a meditative element that calms the nerves, and the movement of the exercises strengthens the muscles. After two stays in our clinic the patient was by and large free of pain. But a mugging on a holiday, which also burdened the patient financially, came as a severe shock—and the fibromyalgia returned. Luckily by then the patient knew how to manage her disease. She fasted once more, performed her exercises regularly, and has been able to reestablish a strong reduction in pain.

## THE PRINCIPLE OF CAUSE AND EFFECT
## IN HORMESIS RESEARCH

"All things are poison and nothing is without poison; only the dose makes a thing not a poison." Paracelsus made this observation in the sixteenth century, and modern biology is now in the process of exploring this concept through research into hormesis.

A medicinal substance is often only beneficial in a very specific dosage—too much of that substance can lead to the opposite of the desired effect and turn the medicine into a poison. Conversely, and this is at the core of hormesis research, small doses of poisonous substances can have healing effects on the body.[22]

Seeing good and bad as two parts of the same thing is something the Western-Christian tradition is unfamiliar with. This duality is more familiar within Eastern philosophy, as seen in the concept of yin and yang being intertwined. Allicin in garlic, curcumin in turmeric, polyphenols and flavone in blueberries—they strengthen the immune system, are anti-inflammatory, antibacterial, and help fight cancer. But in larger quantities they also might be poisonous to the human body.[23]

Hormesis is at the core of the stimulus-response principle of naturopathy. For example, radiation damages cells, but small doses (low-level radiation) activate our repair mechanisms to such an extent that it can be used to treat rheumatism and arthritis.[24] And the right dose of dirt and bacteria, like you might experience living on a farm, doesn't make children sick but protects them from allergies—because their immune systems are kept on their toes.[25]

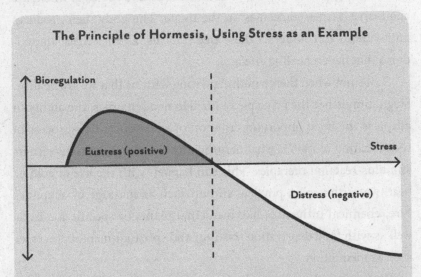

**The Principle of Hormesis, Using Stress as an Example**

Bioregulation

Eustress (positive)

Stress

Distress (negative)

Our bodies are masters of adaptability (bioregulation). We can thus experience low doses of stress as stimulating and even invigorating (i.e., positive stress—eustress). But when stress is unrelenting and there is no period of relaxation, our bodies become overwhelmed and bioregulation is thrown off balance. That's when stress has a weakening and sickening effect (i.e., negative stress—distress).

## WHY MORE HEALTHY THINGS DON'T LEAD TO BETTER HEALTH

There is nothing that is "nothing but healthy." Linearity is not a principle of life. What that means is that more "healthy" things don't necessarily lead to better health. For example, hyperthermia, a

naturopathic therapy that is used to treat cancer as well as fibromyalgia, causes the body to reach high temperatures. This high temperature induces a stress response within the body, causing cells to produce
heat shock proteins, which have a protective effect. Similarly, when
you apply capsaicin, an alkaloid contained in chili peppers, to the
skin, the slight stress leads to the creation of free radicals, which are
aggressive oxygen molecules, in the tissue. The body then produces
antioxidants to counteract these free radicals, and it's these antioxidants that have a healing effect.

So it's not when there's nothing wrong with us that we are healthy.
Stagnation is not the principle of life. Homeodynamics, the ability to
adapt, is the most important criterion of well-being. This process of
reciprocating motion is what naturopathy is trying to initiate with its
stimulus-reaction therapies. This can happen with the use of cold or
heat, water therapies, physical stimuli such as massage or acupuncture, chemical influences like medicinal plants or specific foods, as
well as with food deprivation (fasting) and spiritual-mental processes
such as meditation.

Research in chaos theory has taught us how the smallest forces can
overthrow complex systems and force them to reorganize.[26] This can
be positive or negative. The body's repair mechanisms can be stimulated in such a way that they don't respond to a specific stimulus with
a single reaction, but rather create a healing effect in other areas in
their abundance. This creates some paradoxical effects: Radon radiation in low doses seems to offer protection from lung cancer. This effect could explain why there are rare cases in which remote metastases
shrink after localized radiation therapy as part of cancer treatment—
this is called an abscopal (untargeted) effect.[27]

A dose of a stimulus can cause completely different reactions in
different tissues. This can be observed with exercise: Exertion leads to
physical stress, body temperature increases, and some tissues experi-

ence a lack of oxygen which leads to the formation of toxic molecules. But processes of protection, repair, and construction are also set in motion. That's why endurance training heightens the body's adaptability and strengthens its health, and why exercise is an effective therapy for almost all illnesses.

## THE BODY'S ABILITY TO HEAL ITSELF

"The physician dresses your wounds. Your inner physician, though, will restore your health." This famous quote by Paracelsus refers to what is behind the stimulus-reaction principle described above: our body's extraordinary ability to heal itself.

Most physicians have witnessed the fantastic regenerative capacity of the body—if they know how to allow it to unfold. One of the most important traits a good internist or general practitioner should possess is not treating every symptom but cooperating with the patient to find out what is really going on within the body and whether medical assistance is even necessary.

Months ago, I was planning on seeing an orthopedic specialist because of a persistent pain in my left knee. But I lacked the time and motivation to actually make an appointment. After about twelve weeks I noticed that the pain was beginning to recede. And after five months the pain was gone. A similar thing happened with a mild case of psoriasis, which runs in my family.

In our hospital, it sometimes happens that outpatients have to wait somewhere between three and six months for an inpatient placement due to the long waitlist. For some of these patients, their problems disappear during that waiting period.

Self-healing powers—the expression sounds slightly dubious, almost "esoteric" in the ears of some of my colleagues. And yet, there is something profoundly scientific behind this phenomenon—our body's adaptability to the complex challenges of evolution. After all, we are exposed to a multitude of potentially harmful bacteria, viruses, terrestrial radiation, UV radiation, fine particulate matter, and chemicals on a daily basis. Our genetic material is constantly activated or muted; during each cell regeneration, our DNA, the carrier of our genetic information, is split into two strands and is replicated. Every second, thousands of reactions taking place within our bodies could potentially go wrong and make us sick. And yet we remain healthy in most cases. Therefore, medical practitioners should maybe ask themselves: What is it, then, that actually *prevents* us from becoming ill?

## A SENSE OF COHERENCE

The American medical sociologist Aaron Antonovsky emigrated to Israel in the 1960s, where he came across a study on women in menopause: 29 percent of the participants indicated that they were mentally stable and healthy—even though they had lived through the horrors of the war.[28] What, Antonovsky asked himself, had given these women their strength? He began to conduct research into the origins of health.

After extensive interviews with patients, he developed a kind of matrix as the basis of health. The criterion of "comprehensibility" emerged as a central condition. The question here is: Can I understand what has happened in a bigger context? Do I have any explanation for what is happening? Knowing the answer to these questions brings relief even when the insight doesn't necessarily lead to a solution. As a second criterion, Antonovsky came up with "manageability"—the conviction that crises can lead to positive developments, or the experience of having already overcome worse. Trust is a very important factor: having faith in another person, one's family, a group, or faith in a higher being. Praying has a calming effect on the body—that's why mantras, i.e., the repetition of religiously or spiritually charged words, are a part of the art of healing in Eastern traditions. Most Indian Ayurvedic clinics have a built-in temple, and patients go there to pray in the evenings, when temperatures are cooling down.

Something that is returning to medicine with increasing vigor as "spirituality" was the third constant in Antonovsky's matrix: "meaningfulness." Nelson Mandela is a good example of this: Twenty-five years of political imprisonment couldn't break him. During that time, he completed a law degree by correspondence course and became politically active immediately following his release. He had a meaningful goal—the end of apartheid and the independence of South Africa—and lived, singing and dancing, to the age of ninety-five. This is about the conviction that there are connections that can neither be planned nor calculated, but that require respect and humility in the face of the unknown.

The convergence of these three matrix factors, their overlapping, is what Antonovsky calls a "sense of coherence," the knowledge of an internal connection accompanied by external support. The stronger the sense of coherence, the more stable one's mental health, which has an immense influence on the body. From these ideas, Antonovsky developed a theory on the question of how health and well-being is actually created—salutogenesis. A salutogenic approach to medicine looks at which factors actually keep us healthy. A focus on salutogenesis is an alternative to conventional medicine's focus on pathogenesis—the origination and development of a disease. Antonovsky's goal was to uncover the factors that keep us healthy, rather than focus on what creates disease. Antonovsky suggested that enhancing and supporting the factors that maintain health and resilience might be as important as eradicating disease itself.

How can we wake our "inner physician"? The relationship between

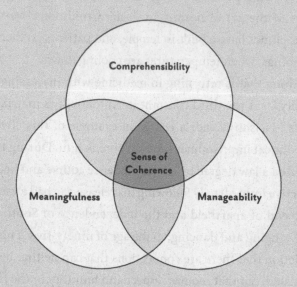

### Salutogenesis: The Origins of Good Health

Comprehensibility

Sense of Coherence

Meaningfulness

Manageability

Health is generated by the interplay of comprehensibility, manageability, and meaningfulness. The intersection of these factors creates a sense of coherence (i.e., knowledge of internal connections accompanied by external support). The stronger the sense of coherence, the more stable the psychological health of a person, which in turn has a major influence on physical health.

doctor and patient is crucial. "Oh well, if we took as much time as the naturopaths," conventional physicians often say, "our patients would be doing better, too." But apart from the fact that we might ask ourselves why we as doctors don't organize ourselves in a fundamentally different way but have created a system of practicing medicine that we no longer consider sufficient and humane, the real secret lies elsewhere: A good physician, I believe, should maintain a sense of equality. It's important never to feel superior to patients, because of our profession and the institution we belong to. I don't treat my patients with condescension. Some doctors think that the need to exude authority is part of the healing effect. But in the majority of cases, the opposite is true. During rounds or in my practice, I am faced with people who are the actual experts, because they know their bodies much better than I do. They know details that can't be garnered from lab results or CT findings. The art of being a physician lies in detecting what has weakened a patient and made him ill, what could be the beginning of the knot, and what could make him healthy again once it is unraveled. Or at least significantly improve his symptoms.

## PLACEBO: THE UNKNOWN POWER OF SELF-HEALING

Naturopathic doctors are often reviled by our conventional colleagues because we make time for our patients. Our treatment methods are often not taken seriously. When our methods work, they're dismissed as "just" the placebo effect, a reaction to the extensive amount of care or a special "setting." Anyone could do it.

The fact is this: What is usually belittled as "imagination" is part of the natural healing process and is connected to the patient's faith that a procedure or a therapy is going to work. When we doctors are able to make a connection with our patients, we create hope and confidence and awake the patient's "inner physician." Neuroscientists like Fabrizio Benedetti have shown how hope activates certain areas of the brain—among other things, oxytocin, a peptide hormone that signals trust, is released.[29] It has also been demonstrated that a painkiller placebo addresses those areas of the brain that are responsible for the moderation of pain just by the expectation of its effectiveness. By using high-resolution MRI scans, doctors at the University Clinic of

Hamburg-Eppendorf were able to show that the body releases opioids that occur naturally—even if the placebo contains nothing but glucose.[30]

As it became clearer that the placebo effect could not be dismissed, a new argument rose in popularity: The idea that it would be unethical to make patients believe they were receiving actual medication. In order to disprove this argument, Harvard professor Ted Kaptchuk conducted the following experiment: In 2010, he openly offered a placebo to patients suffering from irritable bowel syndrome. He explained to patients that the drug contained no active pharmaceutical ingredients, but still worked for many people. And indeed, the group that had taken the placebo performed significantly better and twice as well compared to the control group that didn't receive any treatment.[31] This demonstrated that the success of a placebo does not necessarily depend on the belief that it is real—it works as long as we're convinced that it works.

Kaptchuk also demonstrated the importance of care in another experiment with irritable bowel syndrome patients: A group of 262 subjects was placed on a waitlist and received no treatment for the time being. A second group received acupuncture without any special attention. A third group, however, was "surrounded by care," according to Kaptchuk. The people placing the needles talked to the patients, showed empathy and understanding, and created physical contact with the patients. The results showed that the more care patients received, the more their symptoms disappeared.[32]

"The placebo effect," says psychologist and behavioral immunobiologist Manfred Schedlowski, "is the activation of the body's natural pharmacy."[33] That's why he urges doctors to make more time for their patients.

In 2015, my research group and I invited Andreas Kopf, head of the Pain Center at the Charité Hospital, to lead a training course on placebos. Apart from his work as a pain therapist, anesthesiologist, and placebo expert, he has garnered a lot of knowledge and experience on shamanic rituals by cooperation with African medical institutions. To begin his talk, he listed the core elements of ritualized therapies conducted by shamans or medicine men in traditional and indigenous peoples: the administration of drugs with a sedative or hallucinogenic effect, the move to an unfamiliar location, the ritual washing, and the changing of the patient's clothes. Then the medicine man enters, wearing a ritual outfit and carrying a unique set of tools.

Does this remind you of anything?

Next, Andreas Kopf introduced the rituals of a modern operation: the sedative drugs, the washing and disinfecting of the location of the operation, the putting of the hospital gown on the patient. Then the patient is moved to the OR, where the surgical team, wearing masks and scrubs, is waiting and preparing the tools.

The placebo effect is one of the most complex phenomena of medicine, and it is still not fully understood. Basically, placebo healing exists—with the exception of the most severe emergencies—in almost every medical field. The more chronic an illness is, the more it is characterized by the experience of pain, the higher the placebo effect is.

## HOW TO DELIBERATELY INDUCE SELF-HEALING

So, what does this mean for naturopathy? Symbols, rituals, and even empathy send signals that can be used in a therapeutic manner. Physical contact alone—in acupuncture, wraps, and massages—has a positive effect in our work, as does the fact that we show great interest in the details of a patient's history and condition, because we want to ensure her understanding and cooperation. This may be the biggest difference between naturopathy and conventionally oriented medicine: We not only look at the objectively measurable data, but also the many subjective details that can be instrumental in the healing process—because this makes the patient feel that she is taken seriously, among other things. This is not a strategic method—I know that a big part of my effect as a doctor depends on whether I can strengthen my patient's faith in herself. A good doctor should also never discount a patient's subjective convictions about her illness or her healing as absurd or unscientific, just because she is not able to explain it in the language of the doctor's learned knowledge or because it doesn't fit with the doctor's own world view.

This does not mean that we don't have to run targeted medical interference—yet, the focus of naturopathy, especially where chronic illnesses are concerned, is on inducing self-healing in a deliberate and controlled manner using sensible therapeutic and lifestyle methods.

# CHAPTER TWO

# Therapies of Antiquity Rediscovered

## Leeches, Cupping, and Bloodletting

For most of us, leeches conjure up feelings of fear and revulsion. The idea of one of these strange creatures attaching itself to you in order to drink your blood is probably quite disturbing. This is a normal reaction. I used to feel the same way. That said, leeches are one of the oldest medicinal products in the world. These tiny but effective animals should not be underestimated.

My first encounter with leeches was in March of 1992. It left a deep impression on me. I had just transferred from the cardiology department at the Humboldt Hospital to the department for naturopathy at what was then the Moabit Hospital in Berlin. That's where I was supposed to admit a new patient, a woman in her mid-sixties. She suffered from such severe osteoarthritis of the knees that she was barely able to climb stairs, and could get into a car only with great difficulty. The attending physician ordered leech therapy for the next day.

I was surprised. I had heard that leeches were used in some areas of naturopathy—usually by alternative practitioners—but at a renowned hospital? I hadn't imagined that I would have to be confronted with disgusting leeches on the second day of my naturopathic training. When the appointed time for the leech therapy arrived, I met the nurse who was already on her way to the patient with a pot full of the little animals. Cheerfully, she asked whether I wanted to apply the leeches (for osteoarthritis of the knees, four to six leeches are placed around the joint). I couldn't bring myself to touch the leeches. To be honest, I was nervous that they would bite me.

Over the next few days, I was astonished to see that the patient, who was much braver than I, was doing fantastically well. But how could that be? How could such a seemingly unscientific, medieval procedure make pain in the knees disappear?

## LEECHES: EFFECTIVE ANCIENT HELPERS

There are indications that leeches were already being used during the Stone Age. They can be found in the cuneiform writings of the Babylonians. The Egyptians of the Pharaonic period recognized the healing effect of leeches. Sanskrit papers on Ayurveda mention them, too— leeches were even bred especially to be used in therapy. The Chinese and the Japanese dried leeches and ground them to a powder to be ingested.[1]

In Europe, leeches were initially only used locally in poisonous animal bites—they were meant to clean poison from the wound. Famous doctors of antiquity such as Pliny the Elder or Galen later used them to treat feverish illnesses, chronic headaches, or arthritis. Leech therapy had a resurgence in popularity in Europe in the sixteenth century, beginning in Renaissance Italy, where the gems of classical knowledge were in the process of being rediscovered.[2]

Treatment with leeches is classified as one of the drainage therapies, as is bloodletting, cupping, purging, and fasting. In antiquity, these therapies mainly served to "boost" that which we nowadays know as metabolism. Back then, the declared goal was the regulation of the humors—a theory that follows humoral pathology, the teachings of the four bodily fluids: yellow bile, black bile, phlegm, and blood. All major healing traditions have explanatory models like this, consisting of forces that should be in a certain balance—even if they carry different names and are described differently. These models are often culturally shaped. Our modern idea of effective medicine and what heals correctly is full of such models, too, including the belief— held too strongly for too many years—that antibiotics, i.e., the wish to eliminate all bacteria, are universally good.

Even though we have no more use for "yellow bile" or "black bile" today, humoral pathology was still a reflection of practical knowledge. The terminology of the four fluids was probably not taken literally: They were metaphors for daily observations made by physicians that served to better categorize the various properties and reactions of people. All traditional medical systems have such basic grids in common. In Ayurveda, it's three constitutional types called *doshas: vata, pitta, kapha.* In Traditional Chinese Medicine it's five elements: wood, fire, water, earth, metal.

In the first half of the nineteenth century, medicine began to disproportionately rely on the principles of humorism. Leeches were used excessively—up to a hundred leeches were used at a time. In addition, they were prescribed for all sorts of ailments—perhaps comparable to the misuse of antibiotics nowadays. In the course of this "bloody phase," the yearly consumption of leeches rose from 33.6 million to 100 million in France between 1827 to 1850. Due to high demand the natural population of the animals rapidly diminished. Leeches were imported from Egypt, Syria, Turkey, Russia, and Central Asia. Breeding facilities were created. Leeches became an important medical commodity.[3] Finally, in the mid-nineteenth century, the famed Charité pathologist Rudolf Virchow showed that illnesses have their origin in somatic cells and are caused by changes in the cells.[4] Bloodletting and leeches were slowly abandoned. The modern world jumped at the new, scientifically founded models of explanation in medicine, at cytopathology and microbiology.

Around 1920, there was a sudden renaissance in the use of leeches. In France, thromboses and the resulting vein inflammations were successfully treated with leeches. At that time, no effective medications existed for those diseases. And there was an interest in leeches in wound surgery and military surgery, since it had been observed that wound healing and circulatory disorders after major surgeries improved after a few leeches were attached.[5]

## WHAT HAPPENS WHEN A LEECH BITES

A leech has a pointed mouth with a small sucker and receptors for warmth, touch, and chemical analysis. When a leech encounters a host with a body temperature between 95 and 104 degrees that tastes of glucose or sweat, and if it then possibly feels the pulsing of a vein, it bites. Leeches have, as we know today, a jaw with 240 razor-sharp, tiny teeth that are attached to three jaw blades. Under the microscope, this forms a heart-shaped image. Once a leech has bitten, a wound in the shape of the star in the Mercedes logo remains due to the typical formation of the three jaws. This wound takes a few weeks to heal, because the teeth have essentially carved themselves into the top layer of skin. Yet this barely hurts, because leeches release numerous locally numbing and pain-relieving substances into the wound when they bite—after all, the leech doesn't want to be found by its host animal or human too soon. The bite is often compared to that of a mosquito's.

For most patients, the aversion to leeches subsides once they experience medical benefits of these small animals. Leeches are not moist and slimy, but warm and soft—and sometimes a little lazy. When they stop drinking, you have to caress them carefully, at which point they wake up and carry on. Leeches are also quite sensitive. They need quiet and dim light, otherwise they become stressed and don't bite or suck. And since they need to be in clean water, many leech therapists swear by using specially chosen mineral water to get the best performance from the leeches. For hygienic reasons, leeches can only be attached to a human once—they can live off one meal for up to two years.

I've only had a leech attached to my arm once, just to give it a try. But if I did show certain symptoms, I wouldn't hesitate to be treated with leeches. Simply by observing the effects of leech therapy, it becomes clear that these animals are symbionts—who don't live at our cost but with us. Their saliva contains numerous compounds that prevent the host from suffering any harm. These substances, which facilitate blood coagulation, use similar signaling pathways to those that are activated for the prevention of inflammation. One of these substances is hirudin, a polypeptide (protein) that is very effective at stopping blood from coagulating—thus prolonging the time during which the leech can consume its food. Hirudin is such a strong anticoagulant that researchers initially hoped to use it to dissolve blood clots like those that occur in heart attacks or strokes. However, the substance derived from leech saliva blocked the entire coagulation system to such a great extent that it led to a dangerous amount of bleeding.[6] This area of research was consequently abandoned by the pharmaceutical industry.

In an unrelated study, scientists at the University of Lausanne were able to show that hirudin is not only the strongest known anticoagulant, but also that it notably reduces inflammation of the joints.[7] There are also other bioactive substances contained in leech saliva, so much so that some call the creatures a "miniature pharmacy." For example, their saliva contains hyaluronidase, an enzyme that helps different pharmacologically active substances permeate deeper into the tissue, such as the joint capsule of a knee joint externally treated with leeches.[8] Swelling at the joints is likely reduced after a treatment with leeches because the lymph is activated from the small local venesection that takes place. Moreover, the bite and suction from the leeches themselves cause neural stimuli that change the perception of pain and "overwrite" it in the brain, so to say—a method of pain management that acupuncture also utilizes.

But we still don't fully understand what exactly happens during leech therapy. Why, for example, do certain patients, depending on the thickness of the connective tissue surrounding the joint, respond to it better than others? And we also don't know why the effect lasts for such a long time, usually up to a few months after the treatment. Surely leeches also evoke a strong placebo effect, called "unspecific" in scientific jargon, because most patients consider them exotic, unusual, and positive—all of which are factors that increase the effect they have. But the results of the research I've done with my group indicate that the purely therapeutic effect is significantly larger than what could usually be expected in a placebo effect.

## THE EFFECTIVENESS OF LEECH THERAPY

I couldn't stop thinking about the many successes in treating osteoarthritis of the knees that I experienced during my time at the Moabit Hospital. Many years later, when I was at the Department for Internal and Integrative Medicine at the University Hospital in Essen, I got the opportunity to do research on medicinal leeches. I wondered if it was possible I was misremembering the effectiveness of the therapy. It's easy to forget treatment courses that weren't quite so successful, and patients whom you couldn't treat effectively often don't return to the hospital—and so they stay out of one's personal focus. I wanted to actually examine the efficacy of leech therapy with a critical eye.

I planned an initial pilot study with a total of sixteen patients who suffered severe discomfort from osteoarthritis of the knees. Ten of them agreed to receiving leech therapy; six preferred the standard treatment involving intensive medical gymnastics, physical therapy, manual treatments, as well as massages. At the beginning of the study we asked all participants to evaluate their pain on a scale from one to ten and to repeat this evaluation daily. They did this up until four weeks after the treatment was finished.

The results were surprisingly conclusive. In the ten patients who received leech therapy, the therapy's effect was so pronounced that their discomfort was reduced immensely. Instead of a seven, they evaluated their pain at a one. The conventional physical therapy also brought relief, but much less so. Subsequently, I wrote a scientific report and sent it to the renowned British journal *Annals of the Rheumatic Diseases*.[9] Its publishers very much wanted a photo of the leech therapy. After I had given it to them, they published it on the front cover. The media response was accordingly big, even though it was just a small study.

I particularly enjoy remembering the first patient of this study, a gentleman well into his eighties, who had been gravely restricted in his mobility because of his knee ailment. He was a little doubtful about this therapy, but he was ready to try anything. I asked him to get in touch one year after the study and was surprised to hear that he was still mostly pain-free at that point. He no longer required a walking stick, which he needed before the therapy. The surgery he had been contemplating before leech therapy—a total endoprosthesis of the knee—was no longer an option on the table.

Since the results of the pilot study were so promising, I made plans for a follow-up study on a larger scale. The second study was designed to have a solid structure with a longer follow-up observational period of three months, extensive questionnaires, and a higher scientific standard. This time fifty-one patients participated. It was determined at random which patients would receive treatment with leeches and which patients, the control group, would receive an anti-inflammatory cream (Diclofenac) to be applied to the skin several times a day for pain relief. The start of the study was widely reported in the media, expectations were high, and in order not to disappoint the patients who were assigned to the control group we gave them the option of also receiving treatment with leeches after the study had been terminated. In research jargon, this is called waitlist design.

The results were impressive. Not only did pain decrease this time, but we were also able to demonstrate continued improvement of knee joint function, and, as a result of these two things, an improvement of the patients' quality of life. This time, the study was published in the American journal *Annals of Internal Medicine*.[10] Even the "Bible" of science, *Nature* magazine, reported on it.[11] Magazines like these, which review studies before publication, are of great importance for international scientific recognition. Of course, where scientific news is concerned, it's also a matter of whether the news can be visualized well. Luckily that was the case for us, because television crews from channels such as the BBC and the Discovery Channel came by to film this exotic therapy in our naturopathic clinic in Essen.

A short while later, another team of researchers at the University Hospital in Aachen conducted an even bigger study on leech therapy in osteoarthritis of the knees.[12] In order to determine the placebo effect precisely—the effect that is only caused by the atmosphere, the doctors' friendliness, and the application of the leeches (independent of the substances they release)—this study was single-blinded. This meant that one group actually received leeches as treatment, the other group received a minuscule cut in the skin and a thick bandage—both groups received treatment with a "dressing screen" in between. The patients in question would not be able to tell who got what, neither from pain nor the puncture site. Not only did the study demonstrate that leech therapy had a strong effect, it also showed that the benefits go beyond the placebo effect: The group that received the leeches did notably better than the other group afterward.

On average, 80 percent of leech therapy patients experience a pain reduction of more than half (60 percent on average), three days after a one-time therapy with four to six leeches on the knee. In more than two thirds of patients, this effect persists for more than three months. Almost half the patients (45 percent) use less pain medication after ten months.[13] Ultimately this means that the effect leeches have—and this should be said quite plainly here—exceeds the effectiveness of all traditional pain-relieving therapies for osteoarthritis of the knees known today by far. In many cases, pain medication can even be discontinued, and side effects can thus be reduced.

**PATIENT HISTORY**

## Arthrosis
*Exercise Can Overstrain the Body*

An active life is healthy, but strenuous exercise also has its price. A forty-three-year-old woman, a former professional athlete who now managed a hotel, visited our clinic. After retiring from her sports career, she had continued to work out a lot. But at some point, her knees began to ache. Soon the pain increased. Neither physical therapy nor pain medication worked. She walked around on crutches for almost half a year. At home she took it easy following her orthopedist's advice, who had recommended rest and elevating the legs. She restructured her job as the manager of a hotel in such a way that she was able to do most of her work at the desk. But the lack of exercise made her nervous. At night, the patient only slept at irregular intervals.

The orthopedist suggested a retrieval of endogenous stem cells, preparing and subsequently injecting them back into the knee so as to cause new cartilage cells to grow—one of the many more recent therapeutic approaches in orthopedics, but with an uncertain success rate. Other conventional treatments involve cortisone injections or knee arthroscopy to remove cartilage. But this carries a considerable risk of infection. Moreover, extensive studies have shown that a knee arthroscopy is no more effective than a placebo procedure.[14] A relative advised the former athlete to exhaust all other possibilities before opting for surgery. That's how she came to us, and to the leeches.

We attached six leeches to her left knee. They were still drinking when the swelling in her joint began to noticeably recede. The wounds kept bleeding for twenty-four hours afterward—but the patient was already free of pain, experiencing no discomfort. The effect usually lasts for three to six months, after which the treatment has to be repeated. This patient was pain-free for almost two years after a single treatment. The leeches' saliva cannot get rid of the arthrosis itself, of course, but it contains pain-relieving and anti-inflammatory substances. Our assumption is that the active ingredients reach the entire area of the joint and its surroundings—ligaments, tendons, and muscles around the bite—so that the patient was able to move more freely immediately after having received the treatment. The animals surely also cause a placebo effect. It does look spectacular, after all, when they attach and drink in the rhythm of the heartbeat.

Today, the athlete goes to the gym three times a week and has become an enthusiastic fan of the leeches: She has sent acquaintances and friends to us—and even her mother. In her sixty-nine-year-old mother, the pain hasn't disappeared completely, but her condition has improved. That's why she is going to come back next spring—to us "bloodsuckers," as she calls us affectionately.

## HOW TO APPLY LEECHES

So how exactly is leech therapy carried out? First, the site that is to be treated should be cleaned with water—and only water—since leeches don't like aromatic substances and disinfectants and won't bite if those are applied. If the skin in the treatment area is cool and pale, the circulation of that area should be increased with a hot bath or hot patches. The leech is then positioned onto the area gently. It's best to do this by hand, while wearing gloves. Forceps should only be used in exceptional cases so as not to unnecessarily torture or injure the leech. To prevent the leech from wandering from the treatment area, a small shot glass or cupping glass can be placed over it. Once the leech has bitten, you leave it undisturbed until it detaches by itself, usually after twenty to sixty minutes.

The wound is then dressed loosely with thick cotton dressing or a large, absorbent compress so that the ensuing bleeding isn't hindered.

The site of the bite should be checked by a doctor the following day. Cooling methods, such as a cold pack or a quark poultice, relieve potential itching or redness.

Leech therapy can be repeated—at an interval of four to six weeks, or when the effect has worn off—and is an effective long-term treatment method for treating arthroses. But if a patient doesn't respond after three treatment attempts, success is unlikely. In practice, treating the affected joints in patients with arthrosis at least twice a year has proven successful.

## RHIZARTHRITIS, TENDINITIS, AND BACK PAINS

There have been other medical successes with leeches: We conducted a study on their effectiveness in the treatment of rhizarthritis—arthrosis of the thumb joint. This ailment affects many people, especially women over the age of fifty. The treatment options are quite limited, usually surgery to preserve function of the joint is required sooner or later. Here, leeches showed a clear superiority to the Diclofenac control group. We were able to publish the results in the renowned journal *Pain*.[15] This heralded a renaissance of an ancient therapy.

Subsequently, we were also able to demonstrate the effectiveness of leech therapy in the treatment of tennis elbow (epicondylitis), a very painful tendinitis that can occur as a result of chronic excessive strain after sporting activities, but that can also be occupational.[16] In 2016, when I was already working at the Immanuel Hospital in Berlin, my group and I conducted a study on the effectiveness of leech therapy in the treatment of chronic lower back pain: The results were published in 2018 in the journal of the German Medical Association (*Deutsches Äerzteblatt*) and again, leech therapy showed a considerable advantage over conventional therapeutic exercise in this common ailment.[17]

But where does leech therapy go from here? The findings of all studies on osteoarthritis of the knees have been summarized in a met-analysis by Gustav Dobos and his team in Essen; these are statistical examinations that calculate procedural differences with the aim of reaching an overall evaluation.[18] In light of this data, which is in favor of using leeches, medical insurance companies should be inclined to cover the funding of this therapy for the treatment of arthroses and pain. In the overall evaluation, leeches have proven to be the best possible pain-relieving therapy for painful arthroses—better than anti-rheumatics, pain medication, or certain surgeries. But despite the scientific evidence available, the prejudices against this "archaic" therapy are hard to overcome. That's why many of my patients are still forced to pay for the treatment out of their own pocket, while the costs of orthopedic injections, arthroscopies, and other technical interventions, which are by no means more effective, are covered. I hope that we can eventually overcome our biases against leeches, so that more of us can take advantage of their incredible healing power.

## CUPPING: A CLASSICAL HEALING METHOD REDISCOVERED

After realizing the efficacy of leeches, I became curious. Could there be something to other "archaic" treatment methods? Cupping, for example? Reports about its positive effect on pain, dizziness, or inflammation of the joints can be found in all traditional healing systems—in Tibetan, Chinese, Indian, Greco-Roman, Arabic, and Medieval European medicine.[19] That said, skeptics of naturopathic methods would argue that a treatment method's long tradition doesn't attest to its effectiveness.

This is a worthwhile question to consider. But I think it is hasty of us to completely dismiss a treatment method when a procedure has endured for such a long time and has a history of demonstrated success in folk medicine. Cupping, in particular, also isn't as implausible as critics say. The operating principle of the cupping glasses is negative pressure, which is caused when the glass cools off or by pumping out the contained air through a rubber ball. The negative pressure lifts the top layer of the skin off the deeper-lying layers, which increases the blood flow locally and stimulates the lymph flow. At the same time, cupping also affects areas that are farther removed through certain neural pathways.

But studies that have systematically tested the potential applications of cupping are still rare. At the Moabit Hospital, a research group headed by Malte Bühring examined the effect of wet cupping.[20] In wet cupping, a small incision is made into the skin before the cupping glass is placed onto it. Over the next ten to fifteen minutes, the glass becomes filled with a mixture of blood and lymphatic fluid. The cupping glasses can be applied to different zones such as the back, neck, or hip. What is fascinating is that a treatment carried out on the shoulder can have an effect on carpal tunnel syndrome (pain in the wrist). But in naturopathy, phenomena like this is not uncommon. Anatomically speaking, such reflex zones, i.e., skin, muscle, and connective tissue zones that span the entire surface of the body, have been proven more than a hundred years ago.[21] So, it is possible to experience pain in the shoulder blade when suffering from biliary colic, or discomfort in the lower back when suffering from inflammation of the bladder. And that's why a treatment at the neck and the shoulder can have an effect on the hands.

Given the connected effects of these reflex zones, I wanted to take a closer look at the issue of carpal tunnel syndrome. The carpal tunnel is a narrow passageway in the wrist, between the carpal bones and connective tissue. Several tendons pass through it, as well as the hand's most important nerve, which controls various muscles and regulates the sensory function of the thumb, the index finger, and the middle

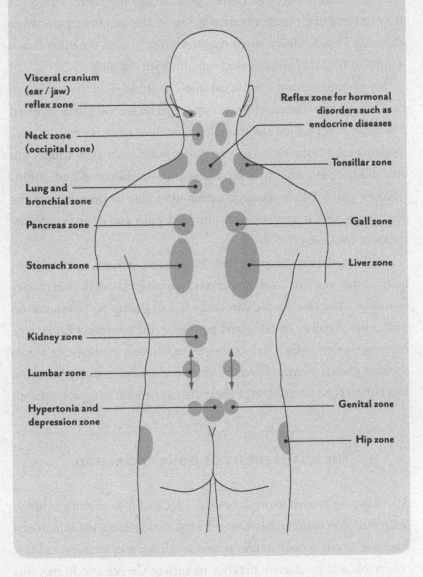

# Reflex Zones for Massage Cupping Therapy

Visceral cranium
(ear / jaw)
reflex zone

Neck zone
(occipital zone)

Lung and
bronchial zone

Pancreas zone

Stomach zone

Kidney zone

Lumbar zone

Hypertonia and
depression zone

Reflex zone for hormonal
disorders such as
endocrine diseases

Tonsillar zone

Gall zone

Liver zone

Genital zone

Hip zone

finger. Injuries, hormonal disorders, rheumatism, or diabetes can cause the tunnel to become narrow and damage the nerve. This leads to symptoms like numbness or tingling in the hands or pain while gripping. This condition often requires surgery. I, on the other hand, wanted to treat this ailment traditionally, with cupping.

My research group conducted another study. The first group of participants was treated with wet cupping. The second group received a pleasant heat pack on the shoulder. One week later, the results were unambiguous: Cupping led to a very clear relief of the symptoms—not only did the pain diminish, but the sensory dysfunction had diminished as well.[22] Other research teams were able to demonstrate the effectiveness of cupping in neck and back pain and even in osteoarthritis of the knees.[23, 24, 25]

Incidentally, dry cupping that requires no incision in the skin is quite simple; you can buy the necessary cupping glasses in pharmacies or online. Any two people can carry out dry cupping treatment on each other. Another relaxing and pain-relieving treatment is massage cupping therapy, which has its origins in Chinese medicine: A single cupping glass is moved over oiled skin in a state of negative pressure. Wet cupping, however, should always be carried out by a professional.

## THE DUAL BENEFIT OF DONATING BLOOD

After cupping proved to be successful, I decided to take matters to the "extreme." Bloodletting has enjoyed a truly bad reputation in modern medicine. Even though there were enough sources that indicated a reasonable and productive practice in ancient Greece and Rome, this practice became widely misused during the eighteenth and nineteenth centuries.[26] Patients were drained of blood at dangerously high levels. A famous victim of this malpractice was George Washington, whose doctors extracted over one and a half liters of blood from him when he had acute laryngitis in 1799, which may have contributed to his death a few days after the procedure. His doctors thought that they could get rid of the "foul fluids" which, in their opinion, had caused the infection.[27]

Did it even make sense to bother examining a therapy of such ill repute in a scientific manner? Well, years before, I had done some research on whether concentrated or less concentrated, i.e., "thick" or "thin" blood influenced a person's health. I noticed that there was a lot to be said in favor of blood thinning, because blood thinning leads to a lower red blood cell count, decreasing the risk of heart attack and stroke.[28] Scientists suspect that menstrual bleeding has something to do with the fact that women who have not yet gone through menopause suffer heart attacks or strokes less frequently than men, though this assumption has never been proven conclusively.[29]

And there were more and more indications that people with excess red blood cells could benefit from bloodletting. For example, in 1991, the hematologist Jerome L. Sullivan published an article entitled "Blood Donation May Be Good for the Donor."[30] I decided to go back to the sources—as I had been taught to do. In the translated writings of the Greek physician Galen, I found clear indications on bloodletting: Patients with a propensity for strokes, who are red-faced and overweight, would benefit from this procedure.[31] I also discovered a doctoral thesis, supervised by Walter Zidek, currently tenured professor for Hypertensiology and Nephrology at the Charité Hospital. This thesis proved that bloodletting can have an antihypertensive effect in people who have undergone a kidney transplant and whose blood pressure cannot be controlled by medication.[32] I contacted my colleague immediately. Zidek confirmed those findings but he also pointed out that he thought the effort it required was too great to treat high blood pressure with bloodletting.

Effort or no effort—on a daily basis, I was confronted with patients who desperately inquired about ways that would make it possible for them to take fewer pills. So, we initiated a study on bloodletting: Sixty-four patients with high blood pressure who were also overweight were divided into two groups. One group received two venesections, four weeks apart, where 13.5 ounces of blood were removed each time (the body contains five to six liters of blood—around 200 ounces). The other group had to wait for this therapy. The results were impressive. Six weeks after the study had begun, the blood pressure in the group treated with bloodletting was already significantly lower than if they had taken certain medications.[33] How was this possible?

To find out, I contacted the hematologist Leo Zacharski, who had conducted a large-scale study on bloodletting in patients with peripheral arterial disease and severe claudication a few years ago.[34] More than 1,200 arteriosclerotic high-risk patients participated in it—some received repeated venesections, others received no additional therapy at all. Zacharski wanted to demonstrate that bloodletting not only improved blood flow, but that it also prolonged the life of these high-risk patients. This, however, only manifested in those participants who were under sixty-five years of age. Still, I was not disappointed with these findings, because even the physicians of antiquity had noted that bloodletting should be considered primarily for younger people.

Leo Zacharski assumed that the antihypertensive effect of bloodletting was not only caused by the reduction of the amount of fluid in the veins, but was also connected to reducing ferritin, a protein that stores iron, in the blood. Studies conducted in Scandinavia have shown that heightened levels of ferritin increase the risk of heart attacks and strokes.[35] We were subsequently also able to show that the antihypertensive effect was connected to lowering the ferritin level.[36]

## TOO MUCH IRON IN YOUR BLOOD IS HARMFUL

Many people who eat an extremely high percentage of meat show severely heightened ferritin levels. But there is also a gene, the hemochromatosis gene, that plays a vital role in people with highly elevated levels of ferritin.[37] This gene is not rare among people of European descent.[38] In its most pronounced expression, this gene leads to severe organic diseases due to the accumulation of iron it causes.

By now it has been proven that elevated iron levels cause increased tension in blood vessels and their inner layers (endothelium) and lead to the increased oxidation of blood fats. When paired with hemochromatosis, a genetic disease, this excess iron can also damage the organs.[39] A team of researchers headed by the endocrinologist Donald A. McClain at Wake Forest School of Medicine was able to show in experiments that an excess of iron reduces adiponectin, a hormone that protects our bodies from diabetes.[40] At the same time, excess iron increases our cells' resistance to insulin, which causes even greater exhaustion of the pancreas. Bloodletting augments the level of this hormone and thus improves sugar regulation. It makes sense, then, that women who have yet to enter menopause are less prone to diabetes and vascular diseases such as heart attacks. After menopause, their risk levels even out at about the same levels as men.

Removing excess iron from the body can possibly protect from cancer. In a long-term analysis of his study five years later, Leo Zacharski found a decidedly lower number of cancer cases in the group that had undergone bloodletting regularly. The astonishing results, published in the *Journal of the National Cancer Institute*, were accompanied by the comment: "The results almost seemed too good to be true."[41]

Back to our own study. After it had been published, I received many letters in which patients reported, among other things, that their blood pressure had always been normal as long as they had gone to blood drives regularly. Hypertension had only developed once their age no longer permitted them to continue donating blood. I still remember one of my own patients who had implored me to perform bloodletting on him since he hadn't been allowed to donate blood in two years. Once he stopped donating blood, his blood pressure started to rise. He had what the physicians in antiquity described as "glut": red cheeks, prone to sweating and overheating. We agreed on a venesection just to see whether it would help and, indeed, his blood pressure lowered considerably.

These results encouraged me. What would it be like, I asked myself, to use blood donation as a form of bloodletting? As early as 1992, this question had been posited by a Finnish research team headed by J. T. Salonen.[42] Why shouldn't you do good and benefit from it at the same time? Wouldn't this be a classic win-win situation?

I contacted Abdulgabar Salama, professor for Transfusion Medicine at the Charité Hospital. Salama had researched the history of Arabic medicine and knew bloodletting from the work of Ibn Sīnā, the legendary eleventh-century Persian physician, also known as Avicenna. Shortly thereafter, we had the chance to work with roughly three hundred patients from the Charité transfusion center. They were advised to come and donate blood according to the legal recommendation, at a maximum of once every three months for women or once every two months for men. Over the course of one year, we closely monitored their blood pressure and other risk factors for cardiovascular diseases. Initially, approximately half of the patients presented with hypertension, so we were interested in how regular blood donation would influence its progression. The result: The higher the blood pressure, the more significantly it was lowered.[43]

We now saw the effectiveness of bloodletting in hypertension therapy. Since there is a shortage of donated blood in blood banks around the globe, it seems to be a good thing to share the potential health benefits of donating blood with donors and potential candidates.

It's possible there is another factor that explains the effect of bloodletting in relation to hypertension. When we donate blood, we stimulate bone marrow, which begins to produce new red blood cells immediately. A normal blood cell lives for about 120 to 160 days. It is not surprising that young blood cells are more supple and flexible than old ones. When we undergo bloodletting, the level of young blood cells rises, and the blood flow works well even in the smallest capillaries. Ultimately, this can also lead to lower blood pressure. And thus, bloodletting is a kind of inherent "fresh cell cure."

There is a lot to discover in the circulatory system: In one study, older mice were transfused with blood from younger mice. Afterward, their decrease in brain function slowed down and atrophying of the nerve cells was retarded.[44] It's presumed that there exists an "aging factor," called $\beta 2$ microglobulin, in older blood, which in this circumstance had been reduced. It's possible this factor could be influenced by bloodletting, but as of yet we are unable to prove it.

Lowering ferritin levels is not suitable for all cardiac patients, especially not for those who suffer from a weak heart. On the other hand, regular bloodletting is helpful in treating a fatty liver, which occurs with increasing frequency and can be quite dangerous. But it's important to remember that bloodletting must not become a substitute for healthy lifestyle choices. For many hypertensive patients, a healthier diet, weight loss, more exercise, and stress reduction should be the most important courses of treatment.

## Stroke Risk
### Gaining from Blood Loss

The patient—a dentist in her early sixties—had landed in the hospital after a stroke scare. She described feeling as though she had "small cotton balls" in her head. Doctors discovered that a large vein in her brain was blocked to a great extent. Her maximum blood pressure reading was at 230 instead of the normal 120.

The dentist was facing stress from all sides: Her practice was facing financial pressure, her husband relegated all household tasks to her, and her youngest daughter was a competitive athlete and had to be accompanied to sporting events. It was all simply too much.

After the stroke scare, the patient stayed in the hospital for a few days. After that, her cardiologist tried to get her blood pressure under control—unsuccessfully. For more than six months, he prescribed different drugs for her to try. Finally, a clinical pathologist at the Charité Hospital advised her to look at the problem in its entirety—and she came to our Department of Mind-Body Medicine.

To lower the dentist's high blood pressure, we performed a venesection: This facilitates the formation of young blood cells that are still supple and glide through the small veins better. Furthermore, this reduces ferritin, which contributes to the hardening of the vascular walls and causes them to become rigid. In two sessions that were six weeks apart, we removed 16.9 ounces of blood altogether. This lowered her blood pressure significantly.

The mind-body team taught the dentist to change her habits. None of us can rid ourselves of stress entirely—but we can make ourselves aware of it and find new ways of dealing with it. It sounds simple, but the dentist had to retrain herself to say no. She reduced her workload by half and employed additional staff. She practiced qigong. Beyond that, the dentist also found the courage to set boundaries between herself and her family. Her husband used to utter remarks like, "Unfortunately, my coat is still at the dry cleaners, because my wife is never here on Thursdays." But by now, her whole family has understood that she needs to put herself first in order to stay healthy. She makes time for herself, pays visits to old friends, and regularly undergoes bloodletting and music therapy.

Now, when she gets stressed out, she resorts to a "quickie"—a short breathing meditation where she inhales, counts backward from ten, and exhales when she has reached one. And if the day was especially stressful, she takes a bath with lavender oil. She can measure how this lowers her blood pressure by ten points straight away. At the moment, it is around 140 / 80 on average. Almost perfect.

## THE ANCIENTS WERE RIGHT AFTER ALL

When I look at studies on the "big three" traditional healing methods—leeches, cupping, and bloodletting—it becomes clear that hundreds of years ago, physicians were already using highly effective methods. It is worthwhile to carefully analyze and examine these traditional methods. The world of science, however, lacks the curiosity to do so—in large part due to a lack of sponsors. The past is often dismissed as old-fashioned or outdated. Leo Zacharski told me that he had very

consciously put the reduction of ferritin in the foreground of his publications: "If you write about bloodletting, you're out," he warned me.
"Nobody wants to hear that." I thought he was exaggerating, but I
found out that he was right. When I submitted my study on bloodletting to journals, I received one rejection after the other. They told me
in no uncertain terms that the scientific data was impressive, but that
they didn't believe that there could be a place for such an "antiquated"
therapy in modern medicine. After I revised the language of the study
to focus on "ferritin reduction" it was soon accepted for publication.[45]

The public, on the other hand, responded in an entirely different
fashion. When we were looking for subjects for our first study on
bloodletting, I found myself buried in inquiries. Ultimately, this
method has found wide acceptance and has established itself as a useful
and promising therapeutic possibility. But I always recommend getting
a physician's consultation and examining your personal results.

CHAPTER THREE

# The Healing Power of Water

*Hydrotherapy*

ydrotherapy—the application of water through various methods, temperatures, and pressures to create a healing effect—
has been a part of my life since I was a child. The town near
where I grew up, Bad Wörishofen, was where Sebastian Kneipp (1821–
1897) made hydrotherapy famous. Kneipp was a Bavarian priest and is
considered one of the forefathers of naturopathic medicine. In the second half of the nineteenth century, as industrialization boomed and
cities began to rapidly expand, many people struggled with physical
overexertion and claustrophobia. Kniepp, known fondly in Germany
as the "water priest," showed people how to regain their inner balance
and restore their health. His trust in the self-healing powers—today
we would call them physical and mental resources—of his patients is
in fact what inspired my own grandfather to become a physician.

Because my father and grandfather practiced medicine in accordance with Kneipp's teachings, Kneipp's hydrotherapeutics were part
of my daily life. My father took morning baths in the small swimming

pool in our garden—even in the icy winter. Life with cold baths and Scotch hose treatments seemed normal to me.

This time was also the golden age of sanitarium treatments in Germany. Across the country, from my hometown of Bad Waldsee to big cities like Essen, there were health resorts and parks with public pools for water treading. Hydrotherapy was practiced and taught from generation to generation. But by the time I was training to become a doctor, things were changing. Hospitals removed bathtubs that had been used for hydrotherapy, and rooms for Kneipp's Scotch hose treatments gathered dust until they were remodeled to house endoscopies, lung examinations, and other functional diagnostic tests.

## WATER: ONE OF THE OLDEST CURES IN THE WORLD

Water is one of the oldest cures in the world. We know that baths were an integral part of day-to-day life in ancient Rome. At the bathhouses, you would begin by entering the caldarium, a room holding hot-water baths. You had to wear wooden shoes to enter the room, since the heated floor reached temperatures of up to 122 degrees. There, you could plunge into tubs filled with hot water. Then, after passing through an intermediate area, you would enter the frigidarium, a cold-water pool in which you would cool off. In the Roman Caracalla baths there are 1,600 marble seats, where people could sit and let themselves be doused with cold water. Sweat baths that didn't use water—similar to modern saunas—and treatment rooms for masseuses and physicians could also be found in the large public baths of antiquity.[1]

Sweat and tub baths have existed in Northern Europe since the Middle Ages—knights and soldiers had brought these traditions home from their crusades.[2] But infectious diseases such as the plague, combined with the Catholic Church's disapproval, caused the baths to slowly be shut down one after the other.[3] In the Baroque age, the healing power of water was rediscovered by two Silesian physicians, Siegmund Hahn and his son Johann Siegmund Hahn.[4] In 1783, Johann Siegmund Hahn wrote the book *Unterricht von Krafft und Würckung Des Frischen Wassers In die Leiber der Menschen, besonders der Krancken Bey dessen Innerlichen und äusserlichen Gebrauch* (*Teachings on the Power and Effect of Fresh Water on the Bodies of Humans, Especially the Sick, in Its Internal and External Usage*), which would later inspire Sebastian Kneipp.

Water is the best medium for transporting heat and cold. Hot stimuli through water relax muscles, stimulate circulation, and raise body temperature. These processes have positive effects on the body—defense cells are activated, and hormones and other messengers are released. Cold stimuli through water, on the other hand, have a pain-relieving and anti-inflammatory effect. As blood vessels contract and the body works to keep its internal temperature up, there is a distinct stimulus-reaction that influences the entire metabolism. For this reason, water treatments where the body is exposed to heat and cold in turns are most effective.

### REDISCOVERING KNEIPP'S HYDROTHERAPEUTICS

Sebastian Kneipp's methods had completely gone out of fashion in the 1980s and 1990s. Many efforts were undertaken to change its image: Portraits of Kneipp were designed in the trendy style of Andy Warhol, and people looked to rebrand it under terms such as "Kneippness," but all to no avail. Kneipp was "out," and he remained so, at least for younger generations. When I used to show images of water treading in my lectures and ask whether anyone knew this therapy, very few students raised their hand.

As costs for water and staff kept rising and insurance companies offered little reimbursement, hospitals and doctors lost money with every Kneipp method they performed, which is why even the last remaining Scotch hose treatment rooms and baths disappeared—except in medical rehabilitation facilities and naturopathic clinics. During my time as a medical resident at the Moabit Hospital, every patient received at least one, ideally two, hydrotherapeutic treatments every day. The same is true at the Immanuel Hospital in Berlin today. We use chest and body compresses; arm, thigh, and knee dousing; foot and full-body baths, as well as various moist wraps, sometimes in combination with medicinal herbs.

In clinical practice, Kneipp's methods have an exceptional effect as supplementary therapies. My very first clinical study dealt with hydrotherapy. Patients with a weak heart (cardiac insufficiency) were instructed to perform Kneipp hydrotherapy twice a day at home, with precise directions on how to perform Scotch hose treatments up to their knees and thighs, and how to apply compresses. The treatments were carried out over the course of six weeks. Half of the patients, chosen at random, were instructed to start this therapy immediately. The other group of patients was advised to perform this therapy from week seven to week twelve. This way, we created two comparable periods of time in each group. We asked patients to report on their quality of life, and we monitored their blood pressure and pulse during exercise on stationary bicycles. During the phase in which hydrotherapy was practiced in the respective groups, patients reported improved quality of life and less discomfort. Patients also had lower increases in heart rate (pulse) while exercising, which is an important indication of successful treatment in cases of cardiac insufficiency.[5] Even though this was a small study, it presented some evidence for the effectiveness of Kneipp treatments.

The positive effect of water, steam, and warmth has also been described by the Japanese scientist Chuwa Tei and his team. In Japan, public baths (*sentōs*) have a long tradition, and special sauna baths (*waon*-therapy) are also used to treat cardiac insufficiency, usually with daily treatments that last fifteen minutes and reach a temperature of 140 degrees. In their study examining the effectiveness of sauna baths to treat cardiac insufficiency, Chuwa Tei and his team showed that heart function significantly improved in patients with cardiac insufficiency because of daily visits to the sauna.[6] The reason is that heat causes blood vessels to widen and blood pressure to lower. The heart is under less strain and shortness of breath improves.

Despite these promising results, hydrotherapy and hydrothermal therapy are not yet established treatments in Western cardiology. Back in 1996, I presented the results of my research on hydrotherapy at an international congress for complementary medicine. When I finished my talk, a British doctor stood up and said, somewhat provocatively, that in England people were also bathing every morning, but no one would think of calling this a therapy. I tried to explain stimulus and reaction, warmth and cold in turns, but I don't think I was successful. And so, Kneipp's hydrotherapeutics remain relatively unknown outside of Germany.

## WHY WARMING YOUR FEET HELPS YOU FALL ASLEEP

If you have trouble falling asleep, have you ever considered the possibility that it might be because your feet are cold? In 1990, a study by Kurt Kräuchi and his team at the University Hospital of Basel proved that this was indeed the case, and the results were published in the prestigious journal *Nature*. When patients' feet were warm, it took an average of ten minutes to fall asleep. But when the feet were cold, it took an average of twenty-five minutes to fall asleep.[7]

The reason for this considerable time difference lies in the way that blood flows to the small blood vessels that supply our tissue, and to the peripheral vessels that affect the cascades of messengers that lull us to sleep. So if you have trouble sleeping, placing a hot water bottle in bed by your feet can be immensely helpful. What helps even more is taking a warm foot bath before going to bed. You can add herbs like mustard flour (careful with the dosage!) or ginger to amplify the effect.

For the general prevention of health issues and for training the immune system, a mixture of warm and cold treatments—cold and hot Scotch hose treatments, baths, or compresses—are far superior to applications that only use warm water. Studies from the 1970s show that in the GDR, where hydrotherapy played an essential role in society, children who visited the sauna regularly were significantly less vulnerable to infectious diseases and missed fewer school days compared to their peers. Scientists have been able to prove that water treading, a simple treatment in which you stand in cold water and walk like a stork (meaning you raise one leg so high that it leaves the water while the other remains in the water), also has positive effects on the immune system.[8] Though it may seem as though water treading in cold water will cool off the feet, it actually has the opposite effect. It warms the feet, because after water treading a physiological counterreaction occurs in which blood vessels in the legs and feet dilate. These signals to the immune system build up protection from common colds.

In Kneipp therapy, as with other naturopathic therapies, the right dosage is critical. People who are especially sensitive to cold temperatures adapt more easily when they receive treatments with warm water only during the first week and move on to interchanging douses in the second week. Close self-observation helps here. Perhaps you have experienced this yourself in the sauna: When you stay in a sauna for too long or go too often, you usually achieve the opposite of the desired effect. The next day, you notice a cold coming on or you feel worn out. The allure of the Kneipp methods lies in the fact that they are suitable for individualized self-application. But this also entails carrying responsibility for your own well-being and taking care of yourself.

## HOW TO USE KNEIPP METHODS IN THE SHOWER

Every morning after a hot shower I perform a full-body Scotch hose treatment with cold water. I start by directing a jet of cold water at my outer right foot, then move upward to the groin, and back down again on the inside of the leg; after that I repeat the process with my left foot and left leg. I use the same principle to treat my arms, followed by circular motions along the chest and face, and finally I douse my back. When I'm tired or exhausted, I stick to a shorter treatment in which I only direct the water up to my knees (this, by the way, also helps with headaches). Kneipp therapies are wonderful preventative healthcare measures and easy for anyone to practice—even children and the elderly.

Study results and clinical experiences have demonstrated to me that Kneipp cures are not at all old-fashioned, but instead a highly topical therapy. Plus, most people love water. My hope is that we can introduce more therapeutic knowledge to public swimming pools and thermal baths because it is definitely not healthy to swim in warm thermal water for an hour or to stay for the fourth *Aufguss** after a stressful day. There is a reason, after all, why attendants in Kneipp saunas have to undergo extensive training.

* When the sauna attendant pours water over heated rocks to increase humidity.

# Full-Body Scotch Hose Treatment

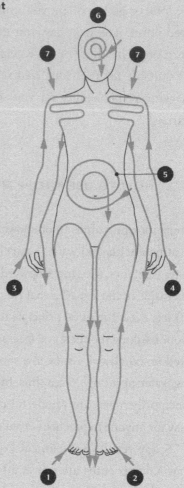

1. Start by positioning the water jet towards the right side of your right foot, then move the water jet up along the outer right leg and direct the water jet over your right buttock and hip and to the inside of the right leg and back down again.

2. Repeat this process on your left leg.

3. Next, the right arm: Direct the water from the back of your right hand upwards to the right shoulder. Let the water flow over the right side of the body, front and back, then move the water downward along the inside of the right arm.

4. Repeat this process with your left arm.

5. Douse your belly with water in a clockwise motion.

6. Douse your face with water, also in a clockwise motion.

7. Finally, pour water over your back.

## The rules are simple:

- Follow these general rules: Right to left, outside to inside, bottom to top.

- Use a jet of water (not a shower).

- For cold water treatment the water temperature should be between 62.6 to 68 degrees Fahrenheit.

- For hot water treatment the water temperature should be between 98.6 to 102.2 degrees Fahrenheit.

- Cold water treatments should only be carried out on warm areas of the skin.

- Keep the treatment short: Stop when you notice a tingling sensation or reddening of the skin.

- Use hot and cold water alternatingly: Start with hot water and finish with cold.

- If possible, don't dry yourself with a towel.

## BETTER RESULTS ARE ACHIEVED WITH WATER
## TREATMENTS THAN WITH DRUGS

At the Immanuel Hospital in Berlin we employ Kneipp therapies as a supplementary method to treat pain, sleep disorders, stress and exhaustion, depression, chronic heart diseases, and circulatory problems. The tremendous effect of water treatments manifests itself particularly when it comes to high blood pressure: In an acute hypertensive crisis, pressure can be lowered in a controlled and effective manner. To do so, the lower arms are immersed in body-temperature water in a sink, then more and more hot water is added until the limit of tolerance is reached, at about 107.6 degrees. This can also be done at home, though you should consult a medical professional about this before trying it in cases of hypertensive crisis.

Using warm and cold water in turns is effective in the long-term treatment of hypertension. Physiatrist Christoph Gutenbrunner at the Hannover Medical School presented an exciting study on the topic about twenty years ago. He observed the progression of blood pressure readings in more than six hundred patients who underwent a Kneipp cure. In people with highly elevated readings, blood pressure sank notably, while it rose in those who had previously presented with hypotension (and who had suffered from circulatory problems as a consequence). The stimulus-response principle had activated the body's self-regulating ability and led to a normalization in different starting conditions.[9] Such an effect that works on two different conditions can never be accomplished by means of a single drug, because drugs only ever focus on one target, one direction.

I highly recommend integrating these pleasant water treatments into your daily routine. You don't need many tools to incorporate them into your life: just a showerhead that can be modified to send out a focused jet of water. Maybe also a bucket, for footbaths. A cold Scotch hose treatment is wonderful in the mornings, after a warm or hot shower. When carried out daily, you'll build a tolerance for the cold water. You might begin by only directing the water up to your knees. Once you're comfortable with this cold stimulus, you can direct the water higher (though if this remains a challenge you don't need to direct the water any higher). At first, it will be difficult for you to direct the cold water to the pelvis and your genital area, or to your back. After a short while, however, you're going to look forward to the invigorating and refreshing effect. The water should ideally be below 64.4 degrees. Dousing your face with cold water is also especially refreshing.

On weekends or holidays, when there's more time available, chest or body compresses can achieve a strengthening and simultaneously relaxing effect. According to our patients, these compresses are among their most impressive experiences. Here, your upper body is wrapped in cold, damp linen cloths, then in a cotton layer, and finally in a woolen blanket. After a few minutes, you'll experience a pleasant warmth. You're stewing in the compresses, in a manner of speaking. But it is important to note that before you start your feet have to be warm, otherwise the desired effect cannot be achieved. If your feet are cold, you can take a warm foot bath or begin with a round of exercise to warm up.

If you have trouble sleeping, a hot foot bath should always be the first step you take. It carries far fewer side effects than medication, and is often successful. Should you have a garden at your disposal, try a dew cure in spring or fall, or treading snow in winter (these are treatment methods in which you go outdoors in snow or while dew is on the ground and walk barefoot for seconds or minutes, until you feel a prickling, sparkling sensation in your feet). Kneipp thought that while doing this, one should imagine that all throughout the night the stars had been shining on the ground.

As harsh as cold stimuli may seem, they are excellent tools for preventative health care: Stimuli and challenges make us stronger! The Genevan philosopher Jean-Jacques Rousseau addressed this in his novel *Emile, or On Education*—walking barefoot, sleeping on a hard bed, hunger, thirst, fatigue, and coldness: All these things can make us tougher. In our affluent society, we can be appreciative of the fact that we are not exposed to these stimuli on an existential basis; and so, it is all the more important to present the body with challenges—always in appropriate doses, of course.

To me, Sebastian Kneipp's hydrotherapeutics are among the most effective therapies that everyone can perform on themselves.

CHAPTER FOUR

# The Value of Restraint

*Fasting as an Impetus for Self-Healing*

A
s George Bernard Shaw once wrote: "There is no love sincerer than the love of food." Few things in life are as satisfying as indulging in a delicious meal. But hunger can and should be your best friend. To explain what I mean, I need to first make a few remarks about the importance of nutrition.

A healthy diet has a significant impact on preventing the major chronic illnesses we suffer from in the Western world, and increasingly in Asia and Africa.[1] We're talking about arthrosis, rheumatic inflammation, high blood pressure, diabetes, dementia, heart attack, stroke, as well as many types of cancer.

Diet and nutrition are immensely important, but it's difficult to get people to commit to eating healthfully. Among experts, the problem is called "delayed gratification." It's hard to say no to someone offering you a cupcake right now, even if you know that it might lead to a stroke in fifty years' time. But believe me: The way you eat now determines whether you're going to spend the latter half of your life healthy or sick.

## PROPER NUTRITION PREVENTS ILLNESS

It can be difficult to properly discuss nutrition because there are so many contradictory statements about what is nutritious. Many lobbyists and pseudo-scientific institutions are involved in funding "scientific" studies and creating the impression that there's no concrete evidence for what is actually, truly healthy. But that simply isn't true.

Considering the entirety of research—experimental laboratory experiments, animal testing, epidemiologic surveys, clinical trials, and experience—there can be no doubt about what constitutes a healthy diet. Each of these five areas of research, however, has its weaknesses. That's why so many results in nutritional research are puzzling and contradictory.[2]

No conclusions about healthy nutrition can be drawn from individual population surveys. Imagine this: On one particular day in a particular year, a patient is asked to fill out a questionnaire about his nutrition. Maybe he hasn't eaten particularly well over the past couple of days and would prefer to forget this fact—and so he fibs. Maybe he generally doesn't pay attention to what he eats or has no idea what's in his meals because they are eaten mainly in restaurants or cafeterias or at home and someone else cooks for him.

In any case, this questionnaire is going to be consulted twenty years later when the patient in question suffers a heart attack and conclusions are drawn as to how nutrition could have been a contributing factor. It's not hard to see how this method is prone to error. But laboratory experiments and animal testing aren't producing unambiguous results, either. From medical research we know that only 10 to 20 percent of drugs that initially test as having positive effects are approved later.[3] Why should this be any different when it comes to nutrition?

And so, we are required to collect all data when it comes to nutrition, including doctors' experience and common sense. Vegetables are very healthy—but have you ever seen advertisements for broccoli in a newspaper or on television? Money is most easily made with fatty, salty, or sweet ready-to-eat foods that beckon with brightly colored packaging. And since a lot of research money is put into these packaged foods, there are studies that are designed to attest to a food product's innocuousness or to some sort of additional functional value. One could argue that Coca-Cola is healthy because it contains a lot of water. So let's go back to the beginning. What kind of diet is actually healthy?

## WHAT HARMS THE BODY MOST IS EXCESS FOOD

I received an answer to this question in March of 1992, on my first day as a medical resident at the Department of Naturopathy at the Moabit Hospital in Berlin. I had come straight from the cardiology department at the Humboldt Hospital in Berlin where we saved lives with heart catheters, the latest drugs, surgeries, and emergency measures—with everything high-tech medicine had to offer. Here, I found myself in an environment that held none of that. The two male patients were having their lunch in a hospital room: One of them was sitting in front of a small bowl of watery vegetable soup, while the other was slowly chewing on a slice of a bread roll, spooning up some milk to go with it. The first one was fasting according to the methods of Otto Buchinger, one of the founding physicians of therapeutic fasting, the other according to the methods of the Austrian doctor Franz Xaver Mayr. Despite the meager meals, the two gentlemen were in high spirits and told me about how their conditions had already improved after only a few days of fasting.

Opponents of fasting argue that it is unnatural. That may be true:

The search for food has been the most important driving force in the history of evolution. But still, fasting has long been a natural part of life: Many animals refrain from eating when they are sick. By doing so, they intuitively contribute to their recovery.[4] And then there are the many animals whose metabolism change as they hibernate. And last but not least, there are millions of people on the planet who regularly practice the art of fasting.

Fasting as a religious practice is almost as old as the history of humankind. Different approaches to fasting are practiced in Christianity, Islam, Hinduism, Judaism (Yom Kippur), and also in Bahaism, Jainism, and many other religions. The Buddha, Moses, and Jesus were said to have each fasted for forty days.

Sometimes medicine is so fixated on scientific data that it is unable to see the forest for the trees. Common sense is enough for us to realize that humankind would have long since ceased to exist if going without food for a few days caused severe health issues. The body has precise programs in place for such times of need—it must be able to regulate temperature, the pH value of blood, or the sugar supply to nerve cells in the brain even under changed circumstances.

Up until the mid-twentieth century, it was more or less a rule of human life that food was not available 24/7. Hard winters and unpredictable circumstances could lead to bad crop harvests. Our body adapted to this regular deficit exceedingly well in its genetic development.

But as exceptional as the body is at handling hunger—due to this long period of adjustment—it has not yet adapted to an excess supply of food. Every year, the number of obese people (men in particular) grows, and there are more and more cases of severe chronic diseases like diabetes and hypertension, as well as cancer and arthrosis. This is not just because we're living longer. Despite all the isolated successes in the fields of cardiology and treatment of hypertension, we have failed at preventative care. About 80 percent of the risk factors for cardiovascular diseases could be eliminated if we ate right, exercised frequently, and avoided a stressful lifestyle.[5]

## FASTING STRENGTHENS IMMUNE DEFENSE

Children possess the natural impulse to refuse food when they are sick, such as with the flu. Parents then often try—with good intentions—to cajole them: "You have to eat, you need to get your strength back!" Scientific studies, however, have shown that fasting during sickness doesn't weaken a person but instead stimulates immune defenses. In 2016, immunologists at Yale University led by Ruslan M. Medzhitov were able to prove that the immune system fights bacteria more efficiently during periods of fasting. This is likely due to the increased number of ketone bodies our body produces when there is a lack of energy, i.e., hunger during fasting. Not so for viruses: Here, the immune cells require energy from glucose to fulfill their defensive function. "Feed a cold and starve a fever," as the saying goes. In short, fasting helps against feverish and purulent infections.

Physicians throughout the ages, from Hippocrates to Kneipp, have observed that refraining from eating—as long as it's not overdone—can promote health. The latter said: "When you notice that you have eaten, you have already eaten too much." When I started to research naturopathic traditions around the world, I observed that fasting is practiced in all cultures. It's fascinating that so many therapeutic methods from around the globe can be strikingly similar, often without the existence of direct contact or exchange. This is similarly true for cupping as a way to treat pain.

The Japanese city of Okinawa is one of the legendary "blue zones" where people on average live to an especially old age. In Okinawa, the rule is that one should only eat until one is about 80 percent full—"Hara hachi bun me." There is a similar saying in Traditional Chinese Medicine: "Chi fan qi fen bao, san fen han"—if you want to stay healthy, you should "only eat until you are 70 percent full and wear only a third of the clothes you would want to put on." In Ayurveda, there is the principle that you should fill one third of the stomach with liquid, another third with food, and leave the rest empty.

## FASTING REGULARLY MEANS LIVING
## A HEALTHIER AND LONGER LIFE

As a resident, I watched as almost all patients with chronic diseases who were admitted to the naturopathic ward of the Moabit Hospital underwent periods of fasting. Among those diseases were, as I mentioned before, diabetes, high blood pressure, rheumatism, enteropathies, and many pain syndromes, in particular migraines, arthroses, and back pain. I quickly realized that therapeutic fasting is much more than just the absence of food. The applied fasting technique is a sophisticated system of specific meals, accompanied by therapies such as liver compresses and Scotch hose treatments as well as baths, exercise, and breathing techniques. Special emphasis was put on the correct way to transition into fasting and then back to normal eating afterward. To transition to fasting slowly and gently, we start with relief days where patients eat fruit or rice to prepare the body and bowel. Fast-breaking correctly is even more important, and involves a careful, step-by-step build-up to meals with a normal number of calories. Patients would often revel in their first bite after fasting, a small ritual celebrated by mindfully chewing freshly cut pieces of apple.

For people who are fasting for the first time, this moment is surprising—how incredibly delicious and stimulating eating a piece of apple can be! This sensation is an important motivating factor for eating healthfully and moderately later on because a good opportunity presents itself after fasting: All senses, particularly the taste receptors, are especially alert and sensitive. Something that may have tasted good before, such as salty sausage or fatty pizza, now seems overly seasoned and hard to digest. Thus, the transition after fasting, which is best done over the course of three days, is very important.

Since I didn't know this when I was a student, my first attempt at fasting—a self-experiment, so to say—went awry. I had decided, with my girlfriend at the time, to undergo a small fasting cure in our apartment in Kreuzberg. We prepared the juices and soups properly. But after the period of fasting ended on the sixth day, we were impatient and celebrated the fast-breaking with pizza. We followed the pizza with cake and coffee. The rest of the day was spent with stomachaches and nausea.

When you look at the tongue, face, and complexion of people who are fasting, you can observe the wonderful effect of this treatment. The facial muscles loosen, connective tissue is drained of excess water, and skin is soothed. In patients with back pain it's possible to see how much the tissue has relaxed by looking at the connective tissue and the back muscles. In many patients, back pain that had persisted for months or even years disappears completely within days.

One should not confuse fasting with dieting for weight loss—weight reduction is only a side effect of fasting. Fasting is not about reducing calories—if you simply eat less, the effect is not the same as fasting. Fasting is about using food deprivation to expose the body to small doses of stress, which leads to a stimulus reaction that detoxes the body and regulates it anew.

Only in recent years has therapeutic fasting finally received scientific recognition. Shortly before December 2015, my colleagues at the Charité and I invited Valter Longo to come to the Max Delbrück

Center in Berlin to deliver a guest lecture. Longo holds one of the most important professorships for gerontology—the study of aging—at the University of Southern California. The lecture hall was packed. Mesmerized, many scientists considered the data presented by Longo. Over the course of many years, Longo had been conducting systematic research on the effect of eating less and fasting in numerous experiments on bacteria, baker's yeast, worms, and rodents. What emerged at the end of this elaborate (due to its many small, isolated parts) research were astonishingly consistent results. His finding was that there is a method by which all living organisms on Earth can prolong their lifespan and remain as healthy as possible while doing so—by fasting at regular intervals or, as an alternative, by refraining from eating one's fill every day and instead reducing the intake of calories by about 20 to 40 percent.

---

**PATIENT HISTORY**

## Rheumatism
*Fasting Changes Lives*

Pale skin; short, dark hair; heavy shadows under her eyes. About fifty years of age, this patient was a doctor herself. Rheumatoid arthritis had attacked her unexpectedly; her slender fingers were swollen and aching. She could no longer perform surgery. Over the course of a lengthy conversation in which her patient history was taken, this woman revealed many worries. She had been trapped in a years-long, expensive divorce battle with her husband. The practice she had opened with another doctor was in a lot of debt. The patient talked about stress, loneliness, and existential fear.

The rheumatologist prescribed the cytotoxin Methotrexate (MTX) and cortisone. Both drugs can be highly effective in treating rheumatoid arthrosis—but for this patient, her condition didn't improve by taking them. She did, however, suffer from the severe side effects the strong medication entailed. That's why she came to our internistic-naturopathic department.

I asked the patient whether she would be willing to fast. She hesitated and asked if that wasn't utter nonsense. She also wasn't sure if she would be able to manage it. Ultimately, though, she was willing to try. After only a few days, the swelling of her hands subsided—a common effect. Her mood improved, which in turn had positive effects on her overall health and well-being.

After completing the fasting cure, the patient completely changed her diet. Today, she only eats meat or fish about once every two weeks. Moreover, she has been seeing a therapist about the conflicts in her life, in particular about the question of what money and her standard of living are worth to her. These conversations can't necessarily solve problems, but they can help patients learn to examine their priorities and reduce the pressure they put on themselves.

The patient's rheumatologist had originally told the patient that she would have to come to terms with the fact that she wouldn't be able to stay in her job for much longer. Her disease was chronic and would only get worse. But things turned out differently. Though she stopped taking the MTX and cortisone, the patient is completely pain-free today. It's only when the stress around her becomes too overwhelming that the swelling of the fingers returns, if only temporarily. That's why the patient made the decision to leave the conflict-ridden practice she shared with

another doctor and to go back to leading her own, smaller practice. Of course, the disease lies dormant within her still, but the
patient has found a way for herself to keep it in check. X-rays of her
joints show no damage today, three years after her first fasting
treatment.

## AN EXPERIMENT WITH A SURPRISING OUTCOME

Valter Longo was mentored by Roy Walford, the very physician and
pathologist who had, together with seven other scientists, lived in a
domed building in the Arizona desert, completely isolated from the
outside world, for two years starting in 1991. The project, "Biosphere
2," which came to international fame, had been financed by an inves-
tor and was meant to test whether an artificially created ecosystem
could sustain itself. NASA supported it, because they thought it might
shed light on whether it would be possible to populate inhospitable
planets like Mars.

But the experiment failed miserably. The concrete construction of
the habitat absorbed oxygen, so air soon became scarce and had to be
pumped in from the outside. Then there were problems with cock-
roaches and spiders. But most devastating of all, the crops of vegetables, fruits, and grains turned out worse than expected. And so, the
first two years of "Biosphere 2" meant two years of hunger for the
participants.[6]

Valter Longo was there when the scientists left the compound,
exhausted and emaciated. Yet even though Roy Walford and his colleagues were only skin and bones, medical examinations showed that
they were not malnourished. Almost all the risk parameters—from
blood pressure to cholesterol levels—had reached an incredibly low

and healthy level. Longo was so impressed that he decided to dedicate his time to gerontology instead of playing jazz guitar (a passion that the two of us share).

After his experience with "Biosphere 2," Walford began advocating a restriction of calories, i.e., a permanent state of slight starvation, as an effective way of reaching one hundred twenty years of age (he himself died at seventy-nine from the genetic disease ALS, which is a considerable age for sufferers from this illness). A community of adherents to this lifestyle was formed, the CRONERs (Calorie Restriction with Optimal Nutrition), some of whom continue to practice the principle of daily calorie restriction, among them Walford's daughter, Lisa. I met her in Mumbai in 2008, at the ninetieth birthday celebration of the Indian yoga guru B. K. S. Iyengar. Lisa is a well-known yoga instructor in the United States and has barely an ounce of fat on her body. On average, CRONERs eat 1,800 calories a day (instead of the standard 2,000 to 2,500 calories).

## THE HEALING EFFECT OF INTERMITTENT FASTING

Calorie restriction, however, poses a number of problems: If you're malnourished for a prolonged period of time, you pay the price of mood swings, a pronounced sensitivity to the cold, and low fertility. The constant reduction of calories is hardly appealing to most people. Malnutrition is a potential problem, and for some strict followers it's possible that anorexia is hiding behind the lifestyle. Valter Longo also realized that a permanent reduction of calories is not a very feasible path. So, he and his colleague Luigi Fontana began looking at alternatives. In experiments involving animals, they showed that it's not necessary to starve oneself constantly. It's enough to fast intermittently. The scientists tested different options, such as the Every-Other-Day

Diet: The test animals, rats in this case, were allowed to eat as much as they wanted for one day. On the next day, they had to fast. The rats would continue eating in this alternating pattern: eating without restriction one day, fasting the next. This caused neither weight loss nor malnutrition, but prevented most diseases of affluence. Not only did the test animals that had to undergo this intermittent fasting not suffer from diabetes or hypertension, they also had very low risk of heart attacks and strokes and were much less affected by neurological diseases such as multiple sclerosis, dementia, or Parkinson's. Their risk of getting cancer was significantly minimized.[7]

## DELIBERATE FASTING IMPROVES CANCER TREATMENT

Back to Valter Longo's presentation at the Max Delbrück Center: What was especially impressive about Longo's data was how it showed that in animals already affected by cancer, the progression of the tumors slowed down when the animals practiced intermittent fasting, and they ultimately lived longer. Longo was careful to emphasize that these findings from experiments on animals could by no means be simply transferred to humans. Yet he did put forward the thesis that chemotherapy and radiation might be more agreeable and less fraught with side effects when accompanied by intermittent fasting. He called this "differential stress resistance."

What does this tell us? Our somatic cells can manage food deprivation well—at least for a certain period of time. These cells possess a centuries-old program that was necessary for survival since food wasn't always available. As a book title by Detlev Ganten, the long-serving CEO of the Charité Hospital, calls it: *Die Steinzeit steckt uns in den Knochen* (*The Stone Age Is in Our Bones*). Taking meals three times a day, perhaps with a snack or two in between, is measured against the long phase of our evolution, a very modern cultural achievement—and very unhealthy.

In evolutionary history, it was the rule that if there was food available, one had to eat it quickly before it perished or someone else came to steal it away. For long periods of time, hunger would be the norm. Winters in particular were barren and were survived by sleeping a lot and eating very little. Our genes, our protein synthesis, and our hormones are, as I have already mentioned, well adapted to this ever-changing program. As soon as energy input by way of food is curbed and this state persists for more than twelve to fourteen hours, our healthy somatic cells begin to enter a mode of protection in which cell growth and metabolic activity are throttled. They enter a state of hibernation, if you will, a kind of standby, which can also protect them like a shield from external attacks such as poisons.

This cell behavior gave Longo the idea to break a taboo: He suggested fasting as a form of cancer treatment. Until then, oncologists had agreed that cancer patients should be safeguarded from weight loss, since weight loss constitutes a bad prognosis in cancer patients. But Longo and his team presumed that during a short period of fasting, healthy cells would actually become more resilient to chemotherapy. This would mean less nausea, less diarrhea, less damage to the nerves, and a higher quality of life.

Cancer cells, on the other hand, are programmed by their oncogenes to grow uncontrolled and uninhibited. Oncogenes are characteristic gene mutations that enable cancer cells to grow fast, without the need for growth stimuli. Unlike healthy somatic cells, cancer cells don't observe stop signals. While the normal somatic cell switches to an ancient protection mode during periods of fasting, the cancer cell "ignores" the state of deficiency and continues to grow unchecked. In this state, the cancer cell becomes particularly vulnerable to chemotherapy, while the healthy somatic cell suffers less damage. Through fasting, chemotherapy and possibly even radiation may become more selective and thus less fraught with side effects.[8, 9]

At least, that's the theory. Whether cancer cells really become more vulnerable through fasting can only be shown after years of research. However, the question of whether fasting makes healthy cells more resilient against chemotherapy was examined in a pilot study by our research team at the Charité and the Immanuel Hospital in Berlin. It started in 2014. We included thirty-four patients who were diagnosed with breast or ovarian cancer and who planned to undergo chemotherapy. Most of them needed to undergo six scheduled treatments. At random, we instructed them to fast for at least thirty-six hours before the start of each of their first two or three rounds of infusion and to eat normally during the other two to three rounds of infusion. With elaborate questionnaires on quality of life and side effects, we gathered information on tolerance to chemotherapy.[10]

The results of our study were consistent with the results of Longo's animal experiments: When they were fasting, patients were better able to tolerate the rounds of chemo and their quality of life was only slightly diminished. During the rounds with a normal intake of food, on the other hand, their condition was worse and their quality of life diminished significantly. In conclusion, many of the patients experienced the positive effects of fasting so clearly that they decided to continue fasting should chemotherapy become necessary again after the study had finished.

Still, the subject of fasting and cancer requires caution. Next, we would like to answer the question of whether fasting actually makes cancer therapy more tolerable in a large-scale study and with the data of one hundred forty patients. More data would help us explore this subject more thoroughly. For example, maybe following a low-calorie diet and refraining from eating animal proteins and sugar has the same effect as fasting during chemotherapy or radiation. Only future studies can provide clear answers.

That said, two initial, smaller pilot studies with humans seemed to confirm Valter Longo's theory. In these studies, Longo's own research team and scientists from Leiden University showed that fasting during chemotherapy makes side effects less severe by ensuring less damage to the genetic substance of somatic cells and impairing blood formation in the bone marrow to a lesser extent.[11] Whether fasting helps the human body fight cancerous cells better can only be clarified in long-term studies.

Specific hormones and foods presumably also play a role in the potential cancer-preventing effect of fasting. Many epidemiological studies attest to the carcinogenic effect of animal proteins.[12] That's why meats and, in particular, sausages were classified as carcinogenic by the World Health Organization in 2015. Numerous animal studies have demonstrated that sulfur-containing animal proteins like methionine and cysteine are carcinogenic—but methionine and cysteine in the body can be reduced by fasting at regular intervals and following a vegan diet.[13]

Sugar also seems to play a significant role in the metabolism of cancer cells. When we cut sugar and quickly resorbable carbohydrates (such as white flour and alcohol) from our diet, we lower the blood levels of insulin and IGF-1, two factors that affect cancer growth. IGF-1 levels can also be lowered substantially through repeated fasting.[14] Additionally, fasting or giving up carbohydrates leads to the production of ketone bodies, which have an anti-inflammatory and antiproliferative effect.[15]

## HOW THE BODY CLEANSES AND DETOXES ITSELF

The positive effects of fasting are thought to be the result of two things that occur in the body: ketone metabolism and autophagy.

When we starve or fast, our metabolism adapts within a few days and slows itself down—it uses less energy. In order to maintain important body functions, we draw upon our body's "storage"—first glycogen in the liver, then fat in the fat stores, and to a lesser extent protein in the muscles and connective tissue. When this happens, our body releases molecules called ketone bodies. Ketones are essentially a second fuel source for cells and the brain. You can detect ketone increase after a few days of fasting by a slight smell of acetone in the breath.[16]

Ketone bodies are also produced during exercise, when fat is burned. Fasting and exercise show surprising similarities here. One of the best ways to prevent degenerative brain diseases like Parkinson's or dementia might be running or walking in a park before breakfast, after fasting overnight.[17] Both fasting and exercise also improve our cognitive ability. Scientists at the University Hospital of Schleswig-Holstein discovered that ketone bodies not only nourish the brain, they also protect the brain from inflammatory cells (which play an important role in degenerative brain diseases).[18]

A prolonged ketogenic diet—a diet in which one eats very few carbohydrates—however, can feel joyless. Even though the ketogenic diet is quite popular at the moment, most people can't imagine a life completely devoid of bread, pasta, rice, potatoes, or sweets. Ultimately, we need proteins and fats to meet our energy requirements. And that's where it's hard to avoid animal products. But in the long run this is counterproductive, because animal proteins are a harmful factor for most diseases of affluence and for cancer.

At the moment, there is some speculation as to whether it's possible to augment ketone balance by consuming coconut oil and palm oil. Coconut and palm oils contain up to 10 percent of medium-chain fatty acids that can be metabolized directly in the liver and lead to the creation of ketone bodies. For a long time, coconut and palm oils were considered unhealthy since they contain a lot of saturated fatty acids, more than butter or meat. But these saturated fatty acids may need to be evaluated differently from a health perspective and might not be as unhealthy as animal saturated fats. Yet whether this outweighs the disadvantages is still questionable. According to most existing studies, the consumption of ample amounts of coconut and palm oils leads to an increase of LDL cholesterol, which is detrimental to a healthy heart.[19] In my opinion, we need to wait for the results of further studies on the matter. At this time, I would not advise consuming large quantities of either coconut or palm oil.

## IT'S NOT ABOUT *WHAT* YOU EAT BUT *WHEN* YOU EAT

When Yoshinori Ohsumi won the 2016 Nobel Prize in Medicine it was a surprise to many, but others thought the recognition was long overdue. Ohsumi, a Japanese scientist specializing in autophagy (from the Greek, meaning "self-devouring"), discovered that somatic cells possess a kind of recycling program that enables them to deconstruct old, damaged, or incorrectly folded proteins into the smallest structures (organelles) and then rebuild them into new complexes. Over years of experiments, Ohsumi was able to show that a cell recognizes when parts of itself have stopped functioning, and that the cell consequently surrounds the nonfunctioning area with a skin (lysosome) and dismantles it piece by piece with the aid of enzymes. This process is initiated in instances where the cell is in distress—during fasting, for example. That's when the cell deconstructs components that have become unnecessary in order to release energy. This energy is then used to form urgently needed molecules. About thirty-five genes control the process of this internal digestion.

Frank Madeo from the University of Graz is one of the world's experts in the field of autophagy. The German-Italian gerontologist has been researching the chains of signals that lead to autophagy in the body. The recycling process, he found, is set in motion when the body isn't producing insulin. The pancreatic hormone that is released after every meal puts a stop to the molecular autophagy machinery.[20]

The biologist Satchidananda Panda at the Salk Institute in La Jolla, California, conducted an experiment on this topic. He fed high-fat food to mice around the clock. The mice developed fatty livers and released high amounts of insulin until their pancreases were exhausted, and they subsequently developed diabetes. During this process, the mice developed the same kind of inflammation that is also involved in arteriosclerosis in the vessels. A second group of mice were fed the exact same number of calories as the mice in the first group—but only over the course of eight hours a day. Surprisingly, those animals stayed slimmer and healthier for much longer.[21]

Findings like these show that it's not only about *what* you eat, but *how* you eat. In his work, Madeo draws the conclusion that we should reduce the number of our daily meals to a minimum—because the cells need time to cleanse themselves. There's not enough time for cells to "cleanse" if the body is constantly releasing insulin as a reaction to food.

As we have seen, a permanent reduction of calories may be joyless, and a meat-heavy ketogenic diet over a long period of time is counterproductive. Research into autophagy and the metabolism of insulin and growth hormones, however, indicates that there's a promising alternative: intermittent fasting. That is, going hungry at regular intervals. By not consuming any calories (including in liquid form) for fourteen to sixteen hours a few times a week, you can achieve a positive health effect.[22]

Autophagy might even contribute to preventing degenerative geriatric diseases. Madeo and his team discovered, rather by accident, a substance that stimulates the cellular cleansing process, even when there is insulin coursing through the bloodstream. This substance is spermidine, a liquid that is found in all somatic cells, but particularly in sperm cells. Spermidine diminishes with age. In elaborate experiments, the scientists in Graz fed yeast cells, and subsequently worms, fruit flies, and mice with spermidine. These organisms lived longer than control groups.

Madeo discovered that spermidine slows down cell aging by stimulating autophagy. In fruit flies, spermidine also increases brain performance. Since in patients with Alzheimer's disease it's the proteins that agglutinate and thus incapacitate nerve cells, scientists are looking for mechanisms that reactivate the cell's cleansing processes—the aim is to use the cell's cleansing process to stop further damage to brain cells.[23] But a lot more research is necessary in order for us to confirm whether spermidine might help the human brain.

## THE TIMING OF MEALS IS THE KEY

The times at which we eat are crucial. In the to-go society we live in, we often don't pay attention to when we take our meals. Yet it is important to not eat uncontrolled all day long, but to restrict yourself to two proper meals a day if possible.

The bowel needs breaks to repair itself: The digestive tract moves in a succession of muscle contractions that extend from the stomach over the entire small intestine and parts of the large intestine in varying phases of intensity. After eating, the gastrointestinal system is inactive so that the food can be macerated. After that, contractions set in at irregular intervals and finally culminate in powerful movements. Like brushstrokes they "sweep" the entire digestive tract in order to cleanse it of food residue. This is called the housekeeper effect. It's this cleaning process that we experience as our stomach rumbles, because air is pressed through the pyloric orifice and causes turmoil. The entire process lasts for up to two and a half hours and is repeated as long as nothing is eaten. The process is interrupted whenever we eat— whether that be treats and nibbles or healthy snacks.

Personally, I try to maintain a period of fourteen hours without any food consumption every day. It's actually not that hard, because I sleep for the majority of that time. Some people omit their dinner; but to me it's important to sit down at the table with my family in the evenings. So instead, I don't eat breakfast and have my first meal at lunch. Until lunch, I avoid snacks and drink a black espresso at most—Frank Madeo, by the way, found out that this increases the level of spermidine in the body—finally some good news on the topic of coffee![24]

## HEALING THROUGH RESTRAINT

The positive effects of fasting begin after a period of fourteen to sixteen hours. You get those positive effects whether you fast consistently every night, or maybe one entire day a week, or seven to fourteen days with medical supervision—as long as you do it right.

I've witnessed the positive effects of fasting time and again, both during my training and in my everyday work with patients. An immediate effect can be observed particularly in cases involving rheumatoid diseases. Fasting as a therapy for rheumatism had already been scientifically proven and published in 1990, but still, to this day many rheumatologists are unaware of it. Instead of using fasting as a supplementary therapy for its anti-inflammatory effect, they prescribe cortisone or antirheumatic drugs like Ibuprofen and Diclofenac to relieve the pain. These drugs do make it easier to live with rheumatism, but over time they produce severe side effects.

A Scandinavian research team headed by the Norwegian physician Jens Kjeldsen-Kragh randomly assigned patients with rheumatoid arthritis into two groups: One group was conventionally treated while the second group underwent a ten-day fasting cure, followed by a vegan and subsequently vegetarian diet. After one year, the second group showed a significant decline in pain, and the swelling of their joints receded, as did joint stiffness. The effect was proven in three further studies, and in 2002, a (summarizing) metanalysis on the subject was published, an important milestone on the path to scientific corroboration.

Studies like these led us to schedule therapeutic fasting as a central therapy during my time as deputy director of the Dr. Köhler-Parkklinik rehabilitation clinic in Bad Elster. Most of the patients there suffered from chronic pain disorders and rheumatic diseases. We recommended a fasting cure for almost everyone. In the neighborhood, we came to be known as the "Fortress of Starvation." When I left the clinic at night to go home, I often saw taxis waiting to ferry our supposedly fasting patients over to restaurants. From witnessing this, I learned that it's crucial a fasting cure isn't prescribed from above but is done voluntarily and carried through by a person's own motivation.

During this same time, I also began to conduct systematic research into therapeutic fasting. Dr. Gustav Dobos and I entered into a collaboration with the brain researcher Gerald Hüther to gain further insight into the role of stress hormones during fasting. Earlier, Hüther had found in experiments on animals that a reduction of food supply over a period of time led to an increased availability of serotonin—the "happiness hormone"—in the brain.[25] I was able to observe this effect in my patients: The first couple of days of fasting were hard on them, and some were plagued by circulation issues or headaches. But after three to four days everyone was in high spirits! Their pulse slowed down and their blood pressure sank—clear signs of relaxation.

I was, however, somewhat baffled when tests of our patients' urine showed that stress hormones also rose during fasting. Nevertheless, the result was unambiguous, and we published it in the journal *Nutritional Neuroscience*. It was only later that science explained this phenomenon with the concept of hormesis. Today I understand that we're dealing with a controlled stress here, a eustress in the original sense of the word, which induces a healthy reaction in the body, as the subsequent work of Longo, Fontana, and Madeo shows in detail.

## THE FASTING CURE IS NOT A DIET

Even though the biological process is called "hunger metabolism," the feeling of hunger is rare in fasting and only occurs during the first two to three days. Moreover, people sleep better while fasting. So fasting, especially under medical supervision, is easier than many patients think.

Some people are concerned about the possibility of fasting triggering health issues. One allegation that is frequently brought up is that fasting damages the heart muscle and causes it to deteriorate. This can be disproven, as the basis for this claim comes from 1960s-era cases in the United States, in which severely obese patients were put on calorie-free diets or diets of protein shakes for several months. Neither things are healthy, and have nothing to do with the fasting cure as practiced by naturopathy.[26]

The second allegation against fasting is the claim of the yo-yo effect, which says that the successes of fasting are nullified because

patients who lose weight would just put the weight back on again afterward. This effect can be seen in many diets that use more or less
arbitrary strategies to reduce weight. Studies show that weight loss diets, no matter what logic they follow, lead to weight gain over a prolonged period of time.[27] But when it comes to therapeutic fasting, this
seems to be different: The observational studies currently available
did not detect a yo-yo effect.[28]

Of course, patients who fast also generally put some of the weight
they had lost back on. This is partly caused by how our tissues—based
on salt intake—store water. During fasting we usually lose one or two
kilos of water, which is essentially "washed out," but which returns to
a certain extent after fasting. Some people also put fat mass back on
again. After the period of calorie restriction the body initially has a
lower demand for energy since it has slowed down many of its "production processes" and the "operating temperature" is also lowered.
So if we subsequently eat with a voracious appetite, the lost pounds
quickly return. But through correctly guided therapeutic fasting, nutritional awareness changes, which is why we don't find any indications of yo-yo effects in our ongoing collection of data. Some of the
people who fast every year reach their initial weight from the year before after twelve months, but this can be classified as a success, because in Europe and the United States it's the rule that we gain weight
every year after the age of forty.

## THOSE WHO PREVAIL REAP SUCCESS

Naturally, willpower is part of fasting. In my native Swabia, Swabian
pockets were invented for the sole purpose of hiding meat in them (to
be eaten surreptitiously) during religious fasting periods. The history
of the art of brewing stouts in monasteries is also related to this

cunning evasion of the dictates of Lent. Human nature reveals itself when it comes to fasting. But by now, plenty of scientific studies have demonstrated the enormous potential of fasting as a therapeutic method. Only ten years ago, I got nothing but condescending smiles from my colleagues when I suggested fasting as a therapy for their patients. Today, I'm met with great curiosity and willingness.

The healing potential of fasting was explored in a documentary called *The Science of Fasting* a few years ago by the French filmmakers Sylvie Gilman and Thierry de Lestrade. They interviewed physicians who specialize in fasting cures as well as patients at the Immanuel Hospital in Berlin. There are about one thousand patients who fast at the Immanuel Hospital every year, but therapeutic fasting has also played a vital role at my previous worksites—the Dr. Köhler-Parkklinik in Bad Elster, the Moabit Hospital in Berlin, and the University Hospital in Essen. Over the years, I've accompanied approximately twenty thousand fasting patients and observed the progress of their illnesses—people afflicted with rheumatism, diabetes, hypertension, and increasingly also with multiple sclerosis and Parkinson's disease, with irritable bowel syndrome, and all sorts of different food allergies.

## IS IT POSSIBLE TO DETOX THE BODY?

When you fast, especially for the first time, you should do so under medical supervision. And even under medical supervision, caution is necessary. Some private clinics earn a lot of money marketing detox cures. I find these practices very troubling. A lot of people have misguided ideas about "toxins." It's always about dosage, about how a substance affects the body, and generally, our body has the ability to deal quite expertly with pesky substances in small doses, as illustrated by hormesis.

But of course, there are a great many environmental toxins, and their negative influence only comes to light when the substances have already been in the environment for a while. We know today that fine particles in the air create a significant risk for cardiovascular diseases.[29] Despite numerous studies conducted on the matter, the question of what amalgam does within the body is uncertain.[30] And without a doubt it's better to limit the amount of pesticides we ingest by opting for organic foods. Just like the pollution of water from lead pipes that we've tried to control, we should refrain from using plastic water bottles if possible. But we can't protect ourselves from environmental toxins completely; they are too widely disseminated already—in the air, the water, and the soil.

But it's possible that for many of those who feel they've been exposed to too many pollutants, it's not actually the substances themselves that are bothering the body, but rather stress, years of maintaining an unhealthy diet, and exercising too little. We know from research on hormesis that small doses of toxic substances aren't necessarily harmful to the body. But where is the individual limit, or at what point are we indeed dealing with a disease caused by environmental toxins? It's difficult to determine this in individual cases, and it's even more difficult to answer the question of whether there is a detox method.

Can we cleanse our body of toxins through fasting? Organic environmental toxins primarily build up in the fat tissue. According to a study from 2011, the concentration of persistent chemicals (POPs, persistent organic pollutants) in the blood of obese people who lose weight increases initially.[31] Whether this has an effect on a person's health is unknown as of yet. What is certain is that, generally speaking, obese people gain a health benefit from weight loss.

## THE BODY'S SELF-REPAIR MECHANISM

We have seen that fasting sets a few things in motion, such as, for example, maintenance processes in the cells. A team from the University of Sigmaringen and the American gerontologist Mark Mattson were able to show that the body's ability to repair itself improved after patients had undergone outpatient fasting therapy over the course of a week: The damages to the genetic material caused by negative influences such as UV radiation or various toxins were repaired more efficiently.[32] A research team headed by Agnes Flöel, a scientist who specializes in researching dementia at the Charité Hospital, was able to show in a smaller study that cognitive and memory functions were improved after a modified fasting method that included liquid nutrition.[33] Maybe this is because more neurotrophic factors are released, or maybe it's that the proteins that build up on the nerve cells like dental plaque on teeth are diminished more vigorously as enzymes increase their activity during fasting.

A few years ago, a research team led by Angelika Bierhaus, who at the time was a professor at Heidelberg University Hospital, published very significant findings on "caramelized" proteins. The technical term for these is "advanced glycation end products" (AGEs). AGEs accelerate arteriosclerosis, heart and kidney diseases, and other processes that are caused by chronic inflammations. We ingest them with our food—they are usually formed during industrial processes in the production of convenience food, when proteins, glycose, and fats are heated up and subsequently consumed. The most well-known of them is acrylamide, which is produced in the process of deep-frying and was first detected in potato chips. But it can also be found in coffee, crisp bread, and cookies, if these have been heated higher than 248 degrees.

These industrially produced AGE proteins are so complex and large that the body is unable to dispose of them with ordinary cleansing mechanisms. It's possible that it manages to reduce them during fasting. Though we don't have definite proof of that, a Japanese research team was able to show in an initial study that AGE proteins are increasingly excreted with urine if a diet that included intermittent periods of fasting was adopted for several weeks.[34]

But what happens when toxins like dioxin, or heavy metals such as lead, mercury, and cadmium that are stored in the fat tissue, are "melted" during fasting? This remains unclear. It is possible they are mobilized and excreted. Maybe they are delivered to the intestine by bile after being mobilized from the fat tissue. This is where the reason for traditional fasting techniques may be hidden: In the Panchakarma cures of Ayurvedic medicine, medicinal ghee and oils are administered, and since the toxins mentioned earlier are liposoluble, you could sequester them that way so that they can be more easily expelled through the intestine. The case could be similar for medicinal clay commonly used in cloister fasting, which also sequesters toxins.

Maybe it's these murky movements of the toxins that are to blame when people who regularly lose or gain significant amounts of weight—i.e., up to thirty-three pounds and more—suffer sudden cardiac death caused by cardiac arrhythmias more often, as the findings of a recent paper presented at a cardiology conference in the United States suggest.[35]

But when fasting is done right, there is no need to worry, since patients do not suffer these extreme changes in weight. Furthermore, many other major factors of heart health, like heart rate (pulse), blood pressure, and the so-called heart rate variability, improve.

## FASTING REGULATES METABOLISM AND HAS
## A STRONG ANTIHYPERTENSIVE EFFECT

One of the most important effects of fasting, as far as we can presently tell, is change in the way hormones are directed. If body temperature lowers, the hormones responsible for metabolic activity, such as insulin or T3, a thyroid hormone, are reduced, as is the level of the growth factor IGF-1. In contrast, there is an immediate increase of the hormones that facilitate urine expulsion, an effect that almost everyone on a fasting cure notices right away on the first day.

Beyond that, we were able to show in our studies that during fasting, a pronounced decrease of leptin, the hormone responsible for regulating fat stores, can be observed.[36] Leptin is a hormone that regulates our appetite and our metabolism, and most of it is produced in the fat tissue. When the body is flooded with fatty and sweet food too often, the cells protect themselves from this excess of energy by developing a resistance to leptin (a similar process occurs with insulin). The cells close themselves off to this hormone. The body then tries to counteract this development and releases more leptin. Unfortunately, elevated levels of leptin and insulin have an adverse effect on the entire body. They contribute to the development of cardiovascular and cancerous diseases.

Through fasting, the whole system is essentially returned to square one. The decrease of leptin and insulin as well as the increased water expulsion probably explain the strong antihypertensive effect of fasting, which we were able to prove in our own studies. In two publications, the American naturopath Alan Goldhamer impressively documented that systolic blood pressure is lowered by up to 30–40 mmHg (millimeter of mercury), which is equivalent to the effectiveness of taking two to three medications (one medication usually lowers BP by 10–12 mmHg).[37, 38] This is why it may be necessary to reduce blood pressure medication before fasting, and sometimes they have to be discontinued completely. After fasting, blood pressure does indeed increase again, but in most cases it does so only up to half of the former reading.

## TREATMENT SUCCESSES IN PATIENTS WITH DIABETES

A severe reduction of calories has a dramatic positive effect on patients with diabetes mellitus—as proven by Sarah Steven from Newcastle University. Of twenty-nine patients who only consumed six hundred calories a day during an eight-week fasting cure, most reached normal blood sugar levels without medication. Fatty livers, a common consequence of diabetes, improved significantly.[39]

Scientists at the Helmoltz Center in Munich and at the German Institute of Human Nutrition (DIfE) in Potsdam found out why: The stress of fasting causes a certain protein to be produced in the liver, which leads to the reduction of fat content in the organ.[40] We often combine fasting with bloodletting in patients with diabetes and/or fatty livers. The latter method has proven to have favorable effects in both diseases, and a combined treatment enhances the healing effect.

Fasting also has a strong anti-inflammatory effect—something that can be demonstrated even on the molecular level. After a rich meal, there is a temporary increase in white blood cells—this is called postprandial leukocytosis, which is the reaction to a slight inflammation that occurs in the cell by the interlinking of molecular processes during the digestion of food. The reverse conclusion is obvious: If every intake of food causes a slight inflammation in the body, fasting should cause a decrease in inflammation. For our body, eating ultimately always entails having to deal with foreign proteins and other foreign substances. The bowel is forced to try and find a compromise—between foreign and toxic substances that have to be expelled, and important substances that are essential for us. All in all, the body can only process food by means of a slight inflammatory and protective reaction. When we fast, this reaction does not happen.

## FASTING STRENGTHENS THE CELL'S ENERGY BALANCE

Oxygen can cause metal to rust. In the body, it also attacks molecules and rips them apart. This is one of the biggest reasons why our cells age. When we eat less or fast, the oxidative stress to our cells is reduced significantly. The less food the mitochondria—our cells' energy plants—have to process, the lower the oxidative stress and the fewer free radicals are produced in turn. Free radicals are chemically highly reactive molecules or atoms. They possess a free electron and, on the search for a partner electron, they can cause damage to other compounds such as proteins or the genetic material, the DNA. For the most part, free radicals in the body stem from mitochondria. That's where sugar and/or fat is converted to energy in the final stage of food digestion. This happens with the aid of oxygen, which can't be entirely controlled. Smoking or exposure to too much sunlight, for example, can cause oxidative stress.

It is essential to reduce oxidative stress in a natural, endogenous way. A lot of people think that it's enough to take vitamin oils or other micronutrients that are advertised as antioxidants. Antioxidants enjoy a good reputation. But the issue is not that simple. The mitochondria and the cells require a certain amount of training. Supplying the body with vitamin pills (advertised as antioxidants) when it is in a state of physical stress, as it is during exercise, for example, is ultimately harmful. The beneficial training effect of exercise on the metabolism is negated. At least these are the results of an impressive clinical experiment conducted by Michael Ristow, an internist and professor for Energy Metabolism at the Swiss Federal Institute of Technology in Zurich.[41]

When the body is exposed to stress, mitochondria are animated to deliver energy—be it for digestion or to fuel a physically demanding activity. During this process, free radicals are produced. But the body is smart. It puts up its defense mechanisms—highly effective endogenous antioxidants. But the body must be able to recognize the need for antioxidants. If we supply our bodies with extra portions of antioxidants from vitamin C, E, or beta-carotene pills, we are likely to prevent the body's antioxidant production process from happening.

This was the starting point for Ristow's study: Participants were asked to undergo an exercise training program over the course of four weeks. Exercise has a positive effect on fat and sugar metabolism, which is why it also helps to prevent diabetes. In the study, the participants who did not take any vitamins, but instead took placebos, had notably better metabolisms. This result calls into question the practice of many athletes who take vitamin pills in the belief that they are increasing their fitness. But in actuality, a great number of free radicals are produced when we perform demanding physical activities. The body reacts immediately by producing more endogenous radical scavengers and initiates more repair processes in the muscle cells and the vessels. But a generous intake of vitamins during training levels out these self-help mechanisms of the body.

This is by no means to say that vitamin pills are always harmful. But it's all about dosage and individual constitution. A sick or very old person who is unable to feed themselves well or whose body shows a lack of self-healing powers may benefit from vitamins. Indeed, there are promising study results regarding the use of vitamins for geriatric or multimorbid people, or patients with advanced cardiac insufficiency. For healthy people, however, the best way to consume vitamins is via the "natural total package," i.e., fruit and vegetables. If it must be pills, I recommend taking only a small amount, twice a week at most. This way, the body's own production of antioxidants isn't massively suppressed.

It's not just exercise that stimulates endogenous antioxidant capacities—fasting does, too. Not only is there less oxidative stress, but for the time after fasting there are more, freshly renovated energy plants—mitochondria—at the body's disposal.

These recent scientific findings allowed me to better understand the results of my first study on fasting, which I had conducted together with Gerald Hüther. In that study, we were surprised to see increases in the production of stress hormones in the body immediately after the start of the fasting period—adrenaline, noradrenaline, and cortisol levels were clearly elevated. There is a simple explanation for this: Fasting does indeed place the body in a state of slight stress in the beginning, because sugar and energy derived from food are initially missing. But the stress hormones kick-start the healthy, endogenous counter reaction. Glycogen stores in the liver are emptied and fat reduction begins. Somatic cells transition quite swiftly to their calmer protective mode, accompanied by a dewatering, antihypertensive effect—which also relieves the intestine—and the increased availability of happiness hormones. That's why our fasting patients were relaxed despite the presence of stress hormones and presented with a slow pulse and low blood pressure.

Moreover, if we fast for longer periods of time or fast on a regular basis, the healthy counter effect becomes even more pronounced. As early as the 1990s, data collected by a research team headed by Lars Göhler at the Charité Hospital was able to prove that the level of stress hormones decreases after about two to three weeks and is subsequently even lower than before the fasting cure was begun.[42] Many fasting patients in our clinic report that the more often they fast, the faster their body enters the mode of relaxation and self-healing.

And so it seems that fasting stress is no different from everyday stress and mental stress. It's always important that the stress is controlled, well-dosed, and self-determined. This kind of stress tends to make us healthy more than anything else, which is true for fasting as well as for exercise, hydrotherapy, and "good" mental stress.

Moreover, fasting leads to an increased production of stem cells. In some of their most recent work, the research team around Valter Longo was able to demonstrate this, a result that once more indicates the regenerative and rejuvenating effects of fasting.[43]

## THE ADAPTABILITY OF INTESTINAL BACTERIA

There are a growing number of studies that connect the microbiome, the sum of our bacteria, to the development and progression of certain diseases. It's become more and more obvious that bacteria in the body—particularly in the intestine—play a role in determining the body's health, for better or worse. The relationship between microbiota (intestinal flora) and the nervous and immune system is essential for the self-regulation (homeostasis) of the body.

There are a confusing variety of organisms living in the intestine—roughly forty trillion bacteria that can be reduced to several main branches and a few hundred species.[44] Which kinds of bacteria colonize us depends on our environment. The path through the birth canal is plastered with bacteria, and infants are exposed to even more kinds of bacteria from the nipples and skin of their mother.[45, 46, 47] Bacteria help us utilize the food we ingest and change their composition rather quickly when we change our eating habits.

If you switch, for example, from an omnivorous diet to a vegetarian one, clear changes in the microbiota can be observed within just a few days. It's difficult, however, to evaluate such changes. What is good, what is bad? What is certain is that diversity of intestinal microbiota is a positive thing. People in industrial countries show a reduced diversity of these tiny helpers compared to people from other parts of the world.[48] After a week of fasting, however, this diversity increases, probably because the restriction of energy supply provides a growth opportunity for different species of bacteria that have, up to that point, only led a marginal existence.[49] Research over the next few years will likely show which changes are caused by fasting and how sustainable they are.

## FASTING PRODUCES FUEL FOR THE BRAIN

I have mentioned ketone bodies several times now. They seem to be pivotal in the health-enhancing effects of fasting. A reminder: During the first twelve to twenty-four hours of fasting, the body makes glycogen reserves in the liver available for the production of energy and sugar. This glycogen is quickly turned into sugar—the brain in particular is in constant need of this nutrient, because its nerve cells are unable to use any other source of energy.

When the glycogen stores are used up, the endogenous fat reduction, i.e., lipolysis, is initiated. The freed fatty acids are used to produce energy. For the brain, however, the body produces a special fuel: ketone bodies. Proteins can also supply a certain amount of energy, but the longer you fast, the more the ketone bodies are called to action.

A ketogenic diet without sugar and carbohydrates is trending at the moment, but ultimately, it's not healthy, because it's difficult to meet the requirements of energy gained from fats and proteins with a vegetable-based diet. But it's possible to increase ketone bodies through intermittent fasting, because the process begins after only twelve to fourteen hours of fasting. It's long since been a well-known fact that ketone bodies have a beneficial effect on nervous diseases. They have been used in modern medicine to treat epilepsy for decades. Even in ancient Rome, people who suffered from severe seizures were locked up and left without food for several days. Back then, it was believed that demons could be expelled that way. But the seizures were probably appeased by the forced production of ketone bodies.[50]

## FASTING MAKES YOU HAPPY

Apart from these physiological markers, it's the effect that fasting has on a patient's psyche that fascinates me especially: From the third to the fifth day onward, most people are in a very positive mood, some are even euphoric—until the end of the fasting period. And such an experience of euphoria has a lasting effect. As a rule, we experience feelings of happiness when we eat a delicious meal, when we are invited to a meal, or when we cook for others. So then why do feelings of happiness and contentedness occur during an ascetic renouncement of food? The answer to this can be found in evolution.

Surely, we wouldn't be populating the planet in such vast numbers if our ancestors, prehistoric humans, had retreated to their caves apathetically and depressed whenever they experienced hunger. Instead, their brain became especially active—a zest for action is probably one of the best ways to ensure a successful hunt for food.

Part of the reason for this emotional contentedness during fasting is due to increased serotonin in the brain. In a study from 1997, Gerald Hüther was able to show that under calorie restriction and fasting conditions, serotonin is released in increasing amounts in the brain.

But there is also an increased production of endorphins, i.e., opiates, in the body during fasting.[51] In addition, one of the most renowned brain researchers and neurobiologists in the world, Mark Mattson, was able to demonstrate in countless experiments in his laboratory that nerve growth factors contribute significantly to brain health and positive mood.[52] The most famous of these nerve growth factors is the BDNF (brain-derived neurotrophic factor). Regular exercise as well as fasting and calorie reduction cause a distinct increase of BDNF levels.

But that's not all: Test animals in Mattson's laboratory that fasted intermittently showed a significantly lower risk of developing Parkinson's disease, multiple sclerosis, or Alzheimer's at a later stage. Even non-avertible genetic diseases like Huntington's disease could be delayed in the test animals by repeated fasting.[53] In a 2016 study we conducted together with Valter Longo's research team and the NeuroCure research team at the Charité Hospital, we were able to demonstrate that therapeutic fasting followed by either a healthy Mediterranean diet or a vegetable-heavy, ketogenic diet could improve the condition and quality of life of patients with multiple sclerosis.[54] In an ongoing study we are examining how this progresses in the long term. All of these are indications that fasting is a promising new treatment method for nervous diseases.

### THE RIGHT WAY TO FAST

Fasting has suddenly become fashionable in the world of medicine, particularly in the United States and Europe. Experts who had been criticizing fasting as dangerous only a few years ago have now switched sides and are in support of fasting. What happened? The shift is due to the impressive experimental data available. I must emphasize here that, even though different ways of fasting have demonstrated excellent effects in animals in lab situations, the results are not so easily transferable to humans. Among other factors, the lifespan of animals is not identical to that of humans. Twenty-four hours of fasting mean something different to a mouse than to a human. So even though it has been shown that intermittent fasting is good for the body, it's much more difficult to say which way to fast is the best.

How should we feel about diets that imitate fasting? Valter Longo has published a tremendous amount of research on the fasting-mimicking diet. We can say with almost absolute certainty that large parts of the positive effect of traditional fasting are due to the fact that sugar (by which I mean not only standard sucrose but also the sugar into which carbohydrates are broken down into) and animal proteins are missing from the food consumed. A second point is that reducing calorie intake by 50 to 70 percent appears to generate most of the beneficial effects of total fasting without the adverse effects. Together with a California company, Valter Longo consequently developed fasting-mimicking dietary concepts for prevention (ProLon) and for chemotherapy (Chemolieve) that include a complete daily package of ready-made food containing about 600 to 800 kcal for four to five days of "fasting." Longo, who donates his profits from these companies to a foundation dedicated to the support of research on fasting, believes that it's only by using such ready-made meals that regular fasting can be accomplished successfully over the entire course of one's life.

Both options are probably important for the integration of the powerful fasting therapy into medicine. For people looking for self-help treatments, traditional fasting might be the preferred way. However, for people who suffer from chronic diseases such as inflammatory, metabolic, cardiovascular, or oncological diseases, a fasting-mimicking diet might be preferable. For people who want to fast on a regular basis for prevention, both options are possible—you can develop a fasting cuisine that caters to your individual tastes or choose the fasting-mimicking diet. Most likely, further fasting-mimicking diets, tailored to a variety of disease states, will be developed by Longo and hopefully reimbursed by health insurance companies in the future.

The hope of enjoying the positive effects of fasting without having to forsake food has yet to be fulfilled. Apart from "imitated fasting" (fasting-mimicking diets), the closest we've come to a drug that mimics the effect of fasting is the diabetes drug Metformin, which, due to its uncertain effect on intestinal bacteria outside of a diabetes treatment, should be considered with skepticism. Resveratrol, a phytochemical derived from the skin of grapes, is also meant to reproduce the anti-aging effect of fasting. But the necessary dosage is high and could not be achieved without other risks—particularly if taken in the form of wine.

## MY RECOMMENDATIONS DERIVED FROM
## MEDICAL EXPERIENCE

Based on naturopathic tradition and my own experiences, it seems best to combine therapeutic fasting under medical supervision or regular cycles of the fasting-mimicking diet with intermittent fasting in everyday life. For example:

- One to two weeks of therapeutic fasting once or twice a year to support the treatment of chronic diseases such as rheumatism, psoriasis, fibromyalgia, diabetes, hypertension, pains, migraines, or irritable bowel syndrome.
- In addition, intermittent fasting in everyday life (also suitable for healthy people as a method of prevention): Omit dinner or breakfast so that you don't ingest any food for a period of at least fourteen hours (that includes not drinking any alcohol). In

general, you should only eat when you are truly hungry. Abstain from having snacks here and there. Moreover, have a day of fasting or cleansing once a week and eat only rice and fruit—but no more than 800 kcal; alternatively, have two such days a month.

Ideally, you should undergo therapeutic fasting in its entirety, by submitting yourself with serenity and concentration. Healthy people should fast anywhere between five and seven days. In specialized clinics, this period can be extended to two to four weeks. The more substantial a person's fat reserves, the easier fasting is for them and the longer they are able to do it. Some people even fast the biblical forty days. Even though some of my out-patients have told me about this euphorically, it seems too risky to me. I would advise against it.

During those days of fasting, you're not on a calorie-free diet. Instead, you ingest about 250 to 400 kcal a day in the form of liquid meals. The most established is the technique according to Buchinger: In the mornings and evenings, you are allowed to drink a small glass of fruit or vegetable juice; at lunch, strained, unsalted vegetable broth. Over the course of the day you should drink two to three liters of liquids, herbal teas, and still water to support the flushing of the kidneys. (I do not recommend drinking coffee or other caffeinated beverages while fasting, as it might lead to stomach complaints.) According to our studies, this is even more effective if you don't drink sweet fruit juice but only vegetable juice so as to achieve a more powerful lowering of insulin and IGF-1 levels. But this can be handled according to individual tastes. In fasting, not everything is beneficial and agreeable to everyone. If, for example, you have a sensitive stomach and the juices cause you problems, you might want to substitute juice with small amounts of oatmeal or rice gruel.

I no longer recommend the classic Franz Xaver Mayr diet, where you eat stale bread rolls and milk. Since more recent studies attest to

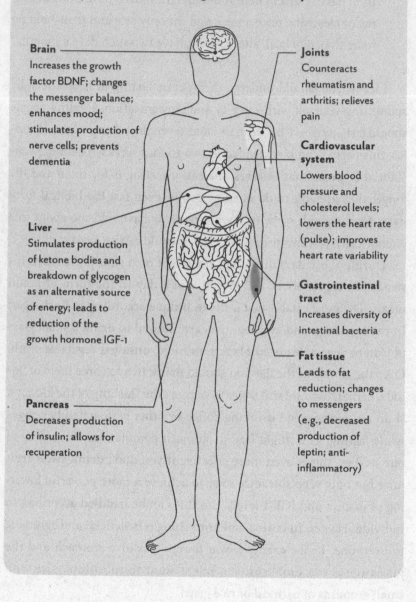

# How Fasting Affects the Body

**Brain**
Increases the growth factor BDNF; changes the messenger balance; enhances mood; stimulates production of nerve cells; prevents dementia

**Liver**
Stimulates production of ketone bodies and breakdown of glycogen as an alternative source of energy; leads to reduction of the growth hormone IGF-1

**Pancreas**
Decreases production of insulin; allows for recuperation

**Joints**
Counteracts rheumatism and arthritis; relieves pain

**Cardiovascular system**
Lowers blood pressure and cholesterol levels; lowers the heart rate (pulse); improves heart rate variability

**Gastrointestinal tract**
Increases diversity of intestinal bacteria

**Fat tissue**
Leads to fat reduction; changes to messengers (e.g., decreased production of leptin; anti-inflammatory)

the fact that omitting animal proteins contributes significantly to the beneficial effect of calorie reduction, it would be paradoxical to drink milk during fasting. Newer variations of the Mayr diet take this into account and substitute dairy milk with almond milk and oat milk.

I do not advise a pure starvation diet, since this facilitates increased and unnecessary muscle reduction.

A lot of patients will tell me about other fasting cures, such as the alkaline diet. This entails several days of eating a vegetarian diet with a lot of root vegetables and no bread. This may certainly be healthy, but it cannot be considered therapeutic fasting because it lacks the essential aspect of reducing calories to less than 500 kcal a day. And this caveat is a major one, because you want to achieve the reduction of endogenous fat and the other beneficial effects prompted by the slight "stress of fasting" on a cellular level. Not only are other new or even traditional fasting methods nonsensical at times, they can also be dangerous. The traditional Schroth cure, for example, consists of taking turns between drinking and dry days, and on drinking days you are encouraged to consume two glasses of wine. At best, this is good for your mood, but not for your body.

It is important to ensure sufficient exercise during fasting. Thereby, the increasing amount of acid that builds up in the body is expelled better through the lungs. There are many more ways in which exercise and fasting complement one another exceptionally well in stimulating cellular repair mechanisms. But it's important to find a good balance between rest and exercise. Some people feel so energetic during fasting that they have no trouble going to work. For others, it's better to visit a monastery, a hotel, or a clinic, and free themselves from all duties and stress (and especially from their smartphone). In general, stress reduction is an essential part of fasting. I thoroughly recommend practicing a relaxation program such as yoga, meditation, tai chi, or qigong during fasting for at least an hour a day.

## ARE ENEMAS NECESSARY?

In the European tradition, each fasting period is meant to begin with a "bowel cleanse": taking a laxative salt such as Glauber or Epsom salts. (As a side note: Since biliary secretions increase significantly during fasting, people with small gallstones should opt for a gentler way to start fasting, with Epsom salts rather than Glauber salts, or a preparation similar to the one used before a colonoscopy. Likewise, people with a predisposition for gout should undergo fasting only with medical supervision.) During the fasting period, it is usually recommended to have an enema every second day. The bowel intensifies its wave-like contractions, its peristalsis, after the intake of food. Everyone has experienced this when the urge to have a bowel movement occurs in the mornings or around noon just after having eaten something. This is called the gastrocolic reflex. During fasting, this intestinal movement is slowed down drastically. With the salts or, alternatively, with an enema, the remains of earlier meals are delivered from the body thoroughly.

There is no data on whether such a procedure improves the success of fasting, medically speaking. Research on this is also influenced by culture. In the United States, for example, people seem to back away from bowel cleanses of any kind because it's such a taboo subject. One disadvantage of emptying the bowel is the loss of minerals and trace elements. I have also observed temporary (benign) dysrhythmias or cramps in the calves. That is why I generally advise a gentle dosage. People with sensitive bowels or who never suffer from constipation and have regular bowel movements don't necessarily need this initial, more intense bowel cleanse. But it's part of the ritual, after all, and it can make the beginning of the fast easier, since it lessens the feeling of hunger. Plus, the feeling of having one's bowels emptied is a pleasant one. The subsequent enemas are appreciated by most people who fast, but in my opinion they are irrelevant to a successful fasting period.

In some fasting clinics, colon hydrotherapies are carried out, where the bowel is cleansed by mechanical irrigation. These are hardly useful. There is no evidence that fasting is improved by this. At most, they provide good additional income to the clinic. The positive results of fasting aren't caused by "flushing away" or "expulsion," but play out invisibly, on the cellular and molecular level.

Midday liver compresses are a powerful supplement to traditional therapeutic fasting: A damp, warm compress in the liver area (applied while resting or lying down for over thirty minutes) improves blood supply to the liver and the gallbladder and intensifies metabolism. Sweating in a sauna or a steam room also supports this process. Blood flow to the skin can be facilitated by massaging the skin with a dry natural hair brush every morning. Similarly, you can brush your tongue (with a toothbrush or a tongue scraper). During my rounds, I see the coating on our fasting patients' tongues change daily. The tongue is a kind of "window" into the intestine—it indicates active metabolic processes. Therefore, cleaning the tongue every morning is useful so you can reduce the bacterial load of the tongue and enhance the cleansing function of fasting. What is not necessary, however, is taking pills or vitamins of any kind. Fasting is holistic and complete all by itself; it does not require any supplementary medication. This also applies to alkaline powders. Alkaline powders can indeed be an appropriate supplementary treatment for chronic kidney diseases, diabetes mellitus, or osteoporosis, since they reduce the acid load that is part of a diet heavy on meat and bread. During fasting, however, the occurrence of acids is a desired part of the transformation process. In a controlled study that I conducted while working in Bad Elster, I compared the overall well-being of one hundred patients who were fasting normally with an equally numbered control group whose participants, in addition to fasting, were given an alkaline powder three times a day. The control group's urine was indeed not as acidic, but otherwise the alkaline powder had no effect on their symptoms and their well-being.[55] Only when a patient suffers from severe back pain or head-aches could alkaline powder or pills be useful, though the headaches that often occur during the first three days of fasting are usually due to caffeine withdrawal. If you drink coffee regularly, you probably won't be able to avoid this annoying initial discomfort.

In any case, you should begin fasting with at least one so-called "day of relief" (with a light meal of unsalted rice) and factor in two days of rebuilding, in which you eat little, light meals, after ending the fasting period. Otherwise you'll render part of the beneficial effect void—just like I did as a student.

## FASTING IN YOUR SLEEP

My advice is to make use of the night. If you sleep from 11 p.m. to 7 a.m., for example, you've already not eaten for eight hours; now you only need another six hours to get to the green zone of fourteen hours. And because it seems like a good idea to not eat too late in the evening, at 7 p.m. at the latest, that's another four hours between your last meal and bedtime. Only have an espresso or some tea for breakfast, maybe a small piece of fruit. Take your first proper meal at lunch. By that time, you won't need to restrain yourself: You can eat until you are full. Your weight may stay the same. However, overweight people tend to lose weight this way. In the United States, this method is also known as "time-restricted eating."

Having said this, researchers disagree on whether it's twelve, fourteen, sixteen, or eighteen hours of not eating that are ideal. Mark Mattson emphasizes that the longer we fast, the more glycogen stores are emptied, and the more ketone bodies are produced: He advises a sixteen-hour fast at minimum, but preferably eighteen hours. Valter Longo advocates the more careful method of 12/12, i.e., twelve hours straight without eating and calorie-intake. He argues that it's harder for people to keep a sixteen-hour break and that they could experience this as stressful, which would then void the positive effect of fasting: "No unhappy fasting!"

The decision is ultimately up to you. Some people may find it easy to cut out breakfast. For others it's no problem to eat as early as 6 p.m. What's important is to test different options so you know which one is right for you.

Fasting requires practice—just like exercise. If you don't feel well after the first two days without breakfast, you should be tenacious and keep going for another two weeks before you draw any conclusions. Only then has the body's metabolism had enough time to adjust. Our internal clock can shift, as it does when you travel to another time zone. The same holds true for daily intermittent fasting. You should be patient but keep listening to your body. But if you still don't feel comfortable after a certain amount of time, you should try something else instead.

## TWO PROPER MEALS, NO MORE

Scientific opinions vary as to how many times a day one should eat. For a long time, it was believed we should have many small, light meals. You can forget that: It's outdated. According to the most recent findings, it's best to only eat two times a day, but have proper meals then. To increase the practicability, Valter Longo allows for another "half" meal, meaning a small portion of a light meal. This, by the way, also corresponds to the recommendations of Ayurveda: In the evenings, you should only have a light, warm soup at most.

One thing is for sure: no snacks in between meals! Even if it's cran-berries or chia seeds. Snacking "to go" has long since become a part of our unhealthy daily routine. Surely, the invention of the snack is re-lated to our packed schedules and the dissolution of our biological rhythms by artificial light, shift work, and other things, with one tricky consequence: fast food instead of slow food. But we doctors aren't completely innocent in this development, either. The disaster probably started with diabetologists. Insulin is a life-saving and ben-eficial therapy for many diabetics. Since it's no simple task to adjust the medication in such a way that there is no danger of hyperglycemia or dangerous hypoglycemia, it was easier to recommend snacks to keep insulin at a relatively constant level and prevent peaks in blood sugar levels.

Today we know that the continuous administration of insulin fos-ters resistance and thus leads to weight gain. Insulin fattens and so it's part of the problem, as obesity leads to further diseases. The legend of the healthy snack is equally as nonsensical as the products for diabet-ics, which were advertised up until a few years ago, which did indeed contain little sugar, but were unhealthy because of their fat content. Then the negative effects of artificial sweeteners came to light along with the fact that they, too, have an effect on the pancreas.

The "to go" trend is supported by the food industry that probably generates more revenue now with a wide variety of snacks. And the problem is evident. Using a newly developed smartphone app, scien-tists Satchidananda Panda and Shubhroz Gill conducted a fascinating study: They asked one hundred fifty citizens of San Diego to take a picture of everything they ate over the course of three weeks. The data was then transferred to the study site immediately, and the details were reviewed. While the majority of participants were convinced that they had relatively regular eating behavior, the data showed an entirely dif-ferent reality: 80 to 90 percent of the participants continuously put something or other in their mouth throughout the day. This kind of unorganized eating behavior equates to pure stress for the body.

In addition, the citizens of San Diego showed a change of behavior on the weekends. On Saturdays and Sundays, meals were taken much later than on weekdays, which is understandable, but for the body it means an exhausting weekly "metabolic jetlag." Afterward, Panda and Gill asked eight of the participants who had never taken longer breaks from eating to eat regularly and to refrain from eating for at least eleven hours at a time, even on the weekends—over a total of sixteen weeks. The results were unambiguous: All participants reported an increase in well-being and improved sleep. Their weight dropped 7.3 lbs. on average without any other dieting. Over the following nine weeks, they didn't put the weight back on.[56]

It no longer seems appropriate for people with diabetes to rely on snacks. Scientist Hana Kahleova at the Charles University in Prague has conducted research on dietary therapies for diabetics. Apart from the advantages of a vegetarian diet for diabetics, she was concerned with the frequency in which meals were taken. By means of a randomized study she put it to the test: Fifty-four patients with type 2 diabetes who were receiving medication were divided into two groups. Both groups received the same number of calories over the course of three months, but the first group was asked to take them in two meals (breakfast between 6 a.m. and 10 a.m. and lunch between noon and four p.m.). The second group took the six meals a day often recommended to diabetics, three bigger and three smaller in-between meals.

The results were clear. After three months, the group that received only two meals a day had lost more weight, and all lab values relevant to diabetes were better in this group. In the two-meal group, fatty livers also improved.[57]

## EAT LUNCH LIKE A KING

This automatically presents us with the question: Which meal should we ideally skip? It's time to question another health myth. Many of us have heard the saying: "Eat breakfast like a king, lunch like a prince, and supper like a pauper." Scientific evidence for the glory of breakfast, however, is scarce. The fact that it curtails the nightly fasting period makes a case against an opulent breakfast. And why is the life expectancy in Mediterranean countries, where people tend to eat rich meals in the evening (which we consider to be unhealthy), longer than in Middle and Northern Europe? Certainly, there are other factors that are of importance here, such as the climate, temperature, and sunlight, that have an influence on the metabolism. When it's warm outside, you feel less of a need to warm yourself up from the inside with the aid of calories.

Instead of breakfast, we should eat lunch like kings. A recently published study attempted to compare a lavish lunch to an opulent dinner. It showed that the participants who consumed the majority of their daily calories at lunch lost weight more easily than those who ate a rich dinner.[58] After all, it's around lunch time that the body requires the greatest amount of energy for keeping its body temperature up— that way, less energy passes into the fat reserves. However, there is a small cultural problem with the issue of an ample lunch. Brain researcher Mattson deducted from his research that it's important for a healthy body to rest for a while to recover after a stimulus like exercise or a big meal.[59] The traditional siesta—a short nap in the early afternoon—has a beneficial effect on a person's health, but it's not feasible in most of the United States, because people's workplaces and homes are too far apart. After all, a siesta shouldn't be taken in a traffic jam on a highway. But if you can arrange for it, if you are working from home, for example, a siesta after lunch is recommended.

Ongoing studies will provide more insights into the optimal timing of meals and duration of the fasting period. Scientists at the University of Padua have presented a study on fasting periods of sixteen hours. They examined thirty-four young, healthy athletes. Half of them were asked to eat three times a day at usual times over the course of eight weeks, the other half were supposed to only eat between the hours of 1 p.m. and 8 p.m. whenever possible. In the latter group, the longer period of fasting led to several beneficial metabolic changes. The blood levels of factors accelerating the aging process, such as insulin and IGF-1, as well as inflammatory factors, were lowered. The sports physician Antonio Paoli and his colleagues observed no such changes in the participants who were adhering to traditional meal times.[60]

A longer nightly fasting period might even be effective in preventing the reoccurrence of cancer, as suggested by initial results of an epidemiological study conducted in the United States. Here, data collected from about 2,400 women with early-stage breast cancer, who had provided information on their eating rhythm at the beginning of the study, was consulted. Roughly four hundred of the participants suffered from new tumors within the study period of seven years. However, women who did not eat for at least thirteen hours after their last evening meal were significantly less affected by recurrence.[61] This was also confirmed by the data derived from animal experiments conducted by Valter Longo, which showed that malignant tissue is unable to cope with a lack of glycose, contrary to healthy tissue.[62] Normal cells have the ability to resort to other energy sources, i.e., ketone bodies, in times of hunger. Cancer cells, on the other hand, do not possess such a hybrid motor and for that reason, they are more likely to perish from a lack of sugar.

If we take a moment to look at the numerous mechanisms that contribute to the protective and healing effects of fasting, it becomes clear that it's much more useful to fast regularly than to exclusively take a specific medication to influence the bodily processes affected by a disease. Of course, statins, the most commonly prescribed lipid-lowering medication, are effective, just as proton-pump inhibitors are used successfully to block stomach acid, or antidepressants are prescribed to treat depressive diseases. But drugs that block individual molecules unquestionably cause dysfunctions in the entire loop system of the body. Usually, little is known about the complex long-term effects of a drug at the time of its approval. The effects only attract attention years later, when millions of people are already taking these drugs.

## FASTING: A WHOLESOME EXPERIENCE

A lot of the time, fasting is defined by the restriction in the number of calories or the supply of nutrients, but this aspect alone falls short. Fasting is a wholesome and, for many people, a spiritual experience. Over the course of our lives, we repeatedly experience deficiencies of some kind—a shortage of money, of success, of affection. Zen Buddhism teaches the "seven hungers" that tempt us to eat even though we are not really hungry: the hunger of the eyes, of the nose, of the mouth, of the stomach, of the psyche, of the cells, and of the heart.

Fasting is a conscious renunciation, a controlled and self-determined experience of deficiency. That's why successful fasting increases self-efficacy—the insight and the motivation that are necessary for us to change our lifestyle successfully. During fasting, we overcome an existential hunger in a way that gives us physical and mental strength. In *Siddhartha*, Hermann Hesse describes this wonderfully: "Nothing is performed by demons; there are no demons. Anyone can perform magic. Anyone can reach his goals if he can think, if he can wait, if he can fast."[63]

# CHAPTER FIVE

# The Key to Health

*Food as Medicine*

When the topic of nutrition is brought up during my rounds, the conversation with the patient usually becomes very lively. Since we all need to eat, nutrition concerns all of us. The World Health Organization estimates that about 50 to 70 percent of chronic diseases can be linked to poor nutrition—an incredibly high percentage.[1] Researchers who deal with prevention have declared that so far, all attempts made to change our lifestyle and our nutritional behavior have failed. These researchers demand stronger directives to be issued by the government, such as printing a traffic-light labeling system (red-yellow-green) on food packaging or imposing a tax on sugary drinks. This may be reasonable, but in my naturopathic opinion, nutritional therapy remains an essential method to bring about change. It is more important now than ever before—we just need to deal with it in a different manner beyond simply counting calories or declaring prohibitions.

It's not all that easy to find legitimate scientific data on which to base medical nutritional recommendations. Studies on nutrition are—since they generally happen in everyday life—much harder to conduct than pharmacological studies, for example, that take place in an experimental setting. Moreover, the industry behind this enormous market keeps trying to deliberately obfuscate or repress data that confirms what has already been known for a long time—that sugar, animal fats, and alcohol are quite unhealthy.

Eating habits are tied to love, comfort, and home—they're habits we don't like letting go of and that are influenced by our culture much more than by logic.

Hardly any other part of our life is so essential to our health, but it is here that medicine is particularly weakly positioned on a professional level. Because who takes care of nutrition? There are dieticians and nutritionists who certainly have a lot of knowledge, but lack day-to-day experience with patients. And so, they end up giving "practical" tips that offer little possibility for implementation. For years, physicians have taken no interest in nutrition whatsoever: Students of medicine learn nothing about it. It was like that when I was studying, and hardly anything has changed today. It is, it must be said, a complete disaster.

This is almost incomprehensible since interest in nutrition is booming. From cookbooks and cooking shows to ever-new dietary trends and countless self-help books, what we eat has garnered a degree of attention that was unimaginable thirty years ago and is already beginning to be annoying. Back then, when I was doing my first internship in the department for internal medicine at the Humboldt Hospital in Berlin, nutritional medicine was more or less dead. At best, there was something like light food for patients who had recently undergone surgery, and diabetics were advised to have snacks and to count calories and bread units (which is completely outdated today). The unanimous opinion of the internists of old was that "no matter what you eat, the most important thing is that the meds are right."

Unfortunately, many physicians still haven't revised their opinion. Time and again, I hear from patients that when they broached the subject of nutrition, their doctor just dismissed the matter. Many doctors do not acknowledge the fact that nutrition can have a very positive influence on illnesses like rheumatism, hypertension, or headaches. As I have already mentioned, it's likely that 50 to 70 percent of diseases are connected to deficient nutrition or have, at the very least, become worse because of it.

Many patients also point out that they don't even know what is healthy anymore, because for years now, media reports on nutrition have been more and more contradictory. One day fat is bad, the next day it's good. One day you're supposed to avoid carbohydrates, but then you're advised to eat whole grains to prevent cancer. A little red wine is good for the heart, but too much is bad, and so on. What's actually true?

## AVOID CONVENIENCE PRODUCTS WHEREVER POSSIBLE

Without a doubt, the food industry and lobbyists of industrial agriculture have massively impinged upon research. In the 1960s and '70s, for example, when it had long since become clear that sugar was unhealthy, leading scientists at the Harvard Medical School were rewarded with bribes for publishing articles in major magazines and indirectly denying facts by cunning omission—today, we would call this "alternative facts."[2] For decades, big corporations like Coca-Cola have been funding and supporting research teams at universities and "independent" institutions that play an authoritative role in the formulation of nutritional recommendations.[3] The meat and dairy industries act with a similarly big influence, especially in the United States.[4, 5] Studies were and are systematically designed in such a way that they deliver as positive a result as possible for these foodstuffs under the guise of "science." Simple methods to achieve this are taking measurements at the wrong time, changing the quantities unrealistically, or providing the control group with worse nutrition.[6]

Neurobiology has shown us that the ample consumption of fatty and sweet foods causes the brain to release messengers signaling rewards that are similarly addictive to hard drugs. This is especially true with combinations of fatty and sweet, like in ice cream.[7] And withdrawal isn't pleasant. Only after a while does it feel glorious to eat without a ravenous appetite and compulsion.

Another issue is that healthy nutrition is often equated with a slimming diet. And so, the question of how obese people can lose weight has been central in past years; 71 percent of Americans are overweight, and of course, losing weight is an urgent wish for many of them.[8] Diets do in fact cause us to lose weight in the short run. But most diets are not actually healthy. One example is the Atkins diet—which asks you to consume a lot of fat, animal proteins, and demands an almost complete refrain from carbohydrates like bread, pasta, or potatoes. Since proteins and fats are saturating and the omission of carbs keeps insulin levels low, you do indeed lose weight quite quickly. But the large quantities of animal proteins and saturated fats expedite atherosclerosis. Put cynically, you'll die earlier, but at least you'll be slim.

Losing weight is not tantamount to becoming healthier. People with normal weight do show a lower risk for cancer in the statistical average, but only if they also exercise and eat healthy. Additionally, people who are slightly overweight and physically active are healthier than slim people who don't exercise.

The great thing about nutritional therapy is that we don't have to take any medication or inject ourselves with something or undergo surgery. Eating in and of itself is not exhausting, and certainly not painful. We don't have to spend any extra time or, if we do it right, any extra money. The only thing that is important is how and what we eat. If you want to interject here that having to eat healthy all the time does indeed hurt your soul, I can comfort you—that feeling goes away. We can change our taste preferences—as it happens naturally over the course of our lives. Do you remember how strange your first sip of beer or wine tasted? Or the first bite of cheese when you were a child? Yet still, we got used to it. I used to enjoy drinking wine, but now I don't drink any alcohol and am doing fine without it.

Most of us don't eat to stay healthy—we eat because things that we have gotten used to due to our culture and upbringing taste good to us. In that sense, changing nutritional behavior is both difficult and easy: For my part, I try to convey to my patients that every habit can be changed.

Each of us has our favorite foods, and if you travel, you'll find that people all over the world claim to have the best cuisine. Genes alone aren't enough to explain such preferences sufficiently. It's our culture and our social environment in particular that seem to be responsible for how tastes are formed.

## DEAN ORNISH, A REVOLUTIONARY CARDIOLOGIST

"Let food be thy medicine" is a claim attributed to the Greek physician Hippocrates, the forefather of medicine. When I began my time as a medical resident in the '90s, this way of thinking about medicine had fallen by the wayside. Therefore, I was all the more impressed by a study conducted by the American cardiologist Dean Ornish, who was a young but already very successful doctor at the time. While doing his training at Harvard, he started having reservations, asking himself whether modern medicine wasn't simply neglecting possible naturopathic courses of treatment.

Ornish himself had grown up doing yoga and was a vegetarian. In an experiment of his that became famous, the "Lifestyle Heart Trial," he put the possibilities of nutritional therapy to the test: He invited severely ill cardiac patients to participate and divided them into two groups at random. One group received the usual cardiological treatment with drugs. The other received very intense and exhaustive training in nutrition and methods of stress reduction. For the participants who, up until that point, had been used to the average American diet containing a lot of meat, Ornish's nutritional therapy meant a radical change. He prescribed them an almost vegan diet, which was also low in fat, for one year—with sensational results: Not only had the participants lost a lot of superfluous weight, their blood cholesterol level and their blood pressure had normalized. But the highlight was that cardiac catheterization showed that the atherosclerosis in the coronary vessels was regressing. In the control group, on the other hand, atherosclerosis, blood fat levels, and hypertension were on the increase over the same period of time. Ornish was able to confirm these results with follow-up examinations five years later and another large-scale study.[9, 10]

In the United States, Ornish's nutritional program is a recognized therapeutic method. The cardiologist has treated many famous patients, such as Bill Clinton, who required stents as well as bypass surgery. When Clinton was facing another surgery, he adopted the Ornish diet, and ever since then he has been slim and much healthier.

Ornish's study has long since become a classic, and to me it remains a milestone. I realized, however, that such a demanding change in eating behavior would be an obstacle to its broad application in medicine. After all, Ornish had been promoting his diet long before plant-based food became a trend and before all physicians were familiar with the term "vegan meals." One challenge was that this diet was meant to be strictly low-fat for heart patients. Even vegetable oils, nuts, or avocados were mostly off limits. But if you consume such a small amount of saturating fats, you have to eat a lot of vegetables to feel satiated.

This was the case for the heart patients I treated with the Ornish diet in the first few years after the study had been published. Many of them got into the habit of carrying some vegetables and other healthy snacks in a Tupperware container to still the rising feeling of hunger. Only later did it become clear that a heart-healthy diet doesn't necessarily have to be low-fat; it's only certain fats that are harmful—others are even important for the vessels' elasticity. But Ornish's diet was successful—and if you keep at it, you do good things for your heart and for cancer prevention. Later, in a different study, Ornish demonstrated that his diet has a positive influence on gene expression—meaning the manner in which the activity of genes is turned on or off—in the prostate tissue of patients with prostate cancer. In this scenario, cancer-facilitating genes were turned off.[11]

### A Healthy Diet, According to Dean Ornish

● ● ● ● ● ● ● ● ● ● ● ● ● ● ● ● ● ● ● ● ● ● ● ● ● ● ● ● ● ●

Our daily nutrition should consist mainly of whole foods: whole meal grain products, raw or boiled vegetables, and fruit. Following this will reduce or even prevent atherosclerosis.

● ● ● ● ● ● ● ● ● ● ● ●

Our daily protein requirement should, for the most part, come from plant sources (e.g., legumes, soy). Dairy products should be reduced as much as possible.

● ● ● ●

Products containing sugar, white flour, or alcohol should make up only the smallest part of our daily nutrition.

## WHAT IS SO HEALTHY ABOUT MEDITERRANEAN FOOD?

Though it is healthy to refrain from eating certain fats, there are plenty of others you can consume instead. This was the surprising message of the first large-scale study on the effects of Mediterranean food on heart diseases, the Lyon Diet Heart Study, which was published by French researchers in 1994. The head of the team, Michel de Lorgeril, from the research center CNRS (Centre National de la Recherche Scientifique), instructed his patients to eat mainly vegetables, fruits, and whole grains. Beyond that, they were allowed to consume plenty of vegetable oils that contain a lot of omega-3 fatty acids, such as canola oil, flaxseed oil, walnut oil, or soybean oil. To make it easier for the patients to consume those fats, a special canola-oil margarine was delivered to their house for free for the duration of the study.[12]

The study was designed to run for a few years but had to be terminated after twenty-seven months for ethical reasons: In the control group, in which patients were eating normally, too many people had suffered a stroke or died compared to the Mediterranean group. The control group was now advised to take up the Mediterranean diet. The data was already sufficient to show that the protective effect of Mediterranean food was great, greater even than that of medications such as beta blockers or ACE inhibitors.

When we hear "Mediterranean diet," we often think of fish, to which many health-promoting qualities are attributed. People who want to eat a healthy diet often replace meat with fish. But fish is far less healthy than most of us probably think. Because fish contains concentrated animal proteins, it creates a lot of acidity in the body, which can contribute to inflammatory diseases, osteoporosis, and arthrosis.

I see an even bigger problem in the ecological question. The recommendation to eat fish regularly lacks a sustainable perspective. Many species of fish are critically endangered, and parts of the world's oceans are overfished. Fish farms aren't a great option because of their use of antibiotics. And many fish are polluted with heavy metals, especially fatty cold-water fish (like salmon or mackerel), which are often recommended for their omega fatty acids.

Fish isn't the decisive health-promoting factor in the Mediterranean diet. The Lyon and the Predimed studies have shown that the beneficial health effects are based on the consumption of olive oil, vegetables, and nuts. The consumption of fish is not relevant. A second misconception is that the long-chain omega fatty acids contained in fish are necessary for treating inflammatory processes in the body, including dementia. Time and again, we hear that plant-based short-chained omega fatty acids are unable to treat these inflammatory processes. But that's not true. It has been proven that alpha-linolenic acid from plants such as flaxseed can, if consumed sufficiently, convert itself into long-chain omega fatty acids.[13] On a side note, algae also provides valuable omega fatty acids. Considering the growing global population, this food source is going to have a bright future. The consumption of algae is probably also one reason why the Japanese are so healthy.

The Lyon, as well as the Predimed study, caused so great a sensation that the Mediterranean diet began its triumphant entrance into medicine. In addition to preventing heart diseases, the Mediterranean diet is also effective against diabetes, rheumatism, hypertension, kidney diseases, and even dementia.

## FOOD IS MORE THAN JUST THE SUM OF ITS INGREDIENTS

Nutritionists as well as many physicians have the odd habit of focusing on the components of food, rather than on the food itself. "Healthy" is not defined by the foods that are actually on the plate, but by the percentage of proteins, carbohydrates, fat, or vitamins the food contains. We're no longer discussing rolled oats, tomatoes, or nuts, but dietary fibers, lycopenes (the healthy pigment found in tomatoes), and fatty acids.

The German chemical scientist Justus von Liebig—who made his contributions during the mid- to late-nineteenth century—is responsible for how food is generally seen as a sum of nutrients.[14] After his colleague William Port had described the three most important components of food—proteins, fats, and carbohydrates (which together are now called macronutrients)—Liebig added a few minerals and declared the mystery of healthy nutrition solved.[15] He then developed a meat extract in the form of stock cubes and the first artificial milk formula for babies (consisting of cow's milk, flour, and potassium bicarbonate). The artificial milk formula in particular shows how simple the idea of nutrition was during Liebig's time. After all, breast milk does not merely contain proteins, fat, and carbs, but also numerous micronutrients and antibodies that have, among other things, an effect on the intestinal flora.

In my view, it was a mistake to divide foods into components: The renowned American author Michael Pollan calls this "nutritionism." In his book *In Defense of Food*, he describes a groundbreaking conference held in 1977: Since the number of chronic diseases was growing at a disconcertingly quick pace, the United States Senate Select Committee on Nutrition and Human Needs issued a recommendation for the "dietary goals" of the United States. Among other things, these guidelines emphasized that the percentage of heart diseases in the United States had increased after World War II, while the rate of this disease was remarkably low in other cultures that traditionally followed a predominantly plant-based diet. U.S. citizens were consequently recommended to restrict their consumption of red meat and milk.

Within a few weeks, however, a storm of indignation—initiated by the cattle and milk lobbies—hit the committee and its chairman, George McGovern. The committee's unambiguous recommendations were replaced by a cunning compromise: "Choose meats, poultry, and fish that will reduce saturated fat intake." Red meat and milk were no longer to blame. The blame had shifted to an anonymous, invisible component, a politically innocuous substance.[16]

Back to the Mediterranean diet: After this particular diet was revealed to be so good for health, researchers began to examine other traditional diets. Studies attested to the health-promoting effects of traditional Japanese or Chinese cuisine.[17, 18] In his best-seller *Blue Zones*, American journalist Dan Buettner identifies "regions of health"—parts of the world where people live longer while staying robust. In addition to the Mediterranean region of Sardinia, there is also the Japanese island of Okinawa, the Nicoya peninsula of Costa Rica, and the stronghold of Seventh-day Adventists, Loma Linda in California. These are also places where the fewest cases of chronic diseases are found.[19]

The common healthy factor that connects the people from these different regions, ethnicities, and cultures is that they all eat a lot of vegetables, fruit, spices, nuts, seeds, and whole grains. For fat, they usually use healthy vegetable oils such as olive oil or nutty fats. Meat is either not eaten at all or only on holidays and/or Sundays.

What the Mediterranean diet has taught us, then, is that approaching nutrition by only looking at macronutrients isn't useful, because not all fats, proteins, and carbohydrates are the same. The Mediterranean diet is not, per se, a low-fat diet. The American psychologist Ancel Keys was one of the first people to research the Mediterranean diet. When he summarized his observations of the eating habits on the island of Crete, he noted that its inhabitants used such enormous quantities of olive oil that you could classify it as a drink.[20] Subsequently, numerous studies have confirmed that fat derived from nuts, soy, canola oil, or avocados has mainly positive effects, while animal

fats, especially those contained in meat, lead to elevated levels of cholesterol, heart diseases, diabetes, and cancer.[21]

One of the biggest studies on nutrition ever conducted made this
point very clear. In the Predimed study, more than 7,500 patients were
divided into three groups at random. One group was prescribed a
Mediterranean diet and was asked to consume 0.26 gallons of olive oil
per week. A second group was also asked to adhere to the Mediterranean diet and eat 1.06 ounces of nuts a day. The third group was asked
to follow a normal, low-fat diet. At the end of the two-year study, the
two groups that consumed large quantities of nuts and olive oil not
only showed lower blood pressure and fewer cases of diabetes, they
also presented with fewer cases of cardiac arrhythmia, depression, and
cancer, and fewer deaths from heart attacks and strokes.[22]

Looking at these extensive nutritional studies, the question of what
constitutes a healthy diet can be answered easily and unambiguously:
We should eat a lot of vegetables, fruits (which aren't as important as
vegetables, however), and a lot of healthy fats from olive oil, canola oil,
nuts (especially walnuts), avocados, and flax and other seeds. Fish is
less important than initially assumed—scientific data does not attest
to a particularly health-promoting effect. And another thing that
unites the healthy diets is that meat makes up only a small part of the
diet or even no part at all. The consumption of dairy products and
eggs is also low.

## HOW UNHEALTHY CARBOHYDRATES PUSHED
## THE SURGE OF OBESITY FORWARD

When I assumed my position as attending physician at the newly-
founded specialty clinic for naturopathy in Bad Elster in 1998, the first
guest we invited was Claus Leitzmann, at the time professor for Nutri-

tional Science at the University of Gießen. Leitzmann had developed a concept called "Gießen Whole-Food Nutrition"—a healthy method for the prevention and treatment of diseases. He had devised two versions: One was strictly vegetarian and the other was predominantly vegetarian but included one meal of fish or meat a week. I still remember his lecture well: "The best meat is the flesh of fruit." There was a controversial discussion on whether animal protein was needed for muscle development, and Leitzmann denied this categorically. His closing comment on the matter was: "Meat *is* not a part of vital energy, it *was* a part of vital energy."

While plant-based fats are predominantly healthy, animal fats are usually harmful. This is partly due to the fact that factory-farmed livestock lead unhealthy and stressful lives and have a bad diet themselves. This has an impact on the meat. When animals are allowed to feed more naturally, for example, when cows can graze in a field, their milk also becomes healthier. The milk of a Swiss Alp cow has a completely different composition than that of a Dutch cow kept in a stable—the Swiss Alp cow's milk contains a lot of healthy omega-3 fatty acids, for example. The Zurich-based cardiologists who conducted this study christened this phenomenon the "alpine paradox": You can eat cheese and stay healthy, as long as you're eating cheese made from the milk of a happy Alp cow.[23]

There's a commonly-held belief that plant proteins have to be combined in complicated ways in order to unfold the same biological power in the body as animal proteins. According to most recent data, this assumption is wrong: The body breaks down proteins and rebuilds them in the way it needs—no matter whether they come from an animal or a plant.[24, 25]

One should also take a differentiated look at carbs. In their natural form found in whole-wheat bread, whole-wheat pasta, or whole-grain rice they sustain health and lower the risk of heart attacks or strokes.

The hitherto largest study overview on this issue showed that the risk of cancer and circulatory disorders is significantly lowered if you eat at least three portions of whole-grain (3.17 ounces), e.g., two slices of whole-grain bread, a day.[26]

Whole-grain products are excellent sources of fiber. They also contain B vitamins and minerals such as magnesium and zinc, because they still hold the sprout, bran, and the outer husks (all of which are removed in ground flour). But the food industry continues to distribute enormous quantities of nutrient-deficient white bread, pasta, and polished rice. Carbohydrates in the form of soft drinks that contain no healthy ingredients whatsoever, and have therefore even been dubbed "liquid candy" in the United States, are the worst.

Breakfast cereals were invented by John Harvey Kellogg, an American doctor and naturopath, with the intention to provide healthy nourishment to the population (which was eating bacon and eggs for breakfast back then).[27] But over time these cereals have mutated into a mixture of unhealthy white flour and lots of sugar, often mixed with artificially added vitamins, since those are lost in the manufacturing process. Even organic supermarkets are selling fewer rolled oats and more sweetened breakfast cereals and muesli bars year by year.

Such unhealthy carbohydrates are likely to have propelled the surge of obesity in Europe and America. White flour is quickly turned into sugar in the body. The body also turns fat into energy quickly. This is why fast food is so problematic: It combines these two negative factors: white flour and fat—for example, donuts, pizza, and burgers. The pancreas then releases huge quantities of insulin—this hormone stimulates fat synthesis and channels nutrients to the cells. This expedites weight gain (which is why insulin is also used to fatten animals). When insulin levels subsequently fall quickly—as the calories have been converted quickly—voracious appetite subsequently occurs. This is not the case with whole grains, because the energy is converted much more slowly. Instead, whole grains stabilize insulin levels.[28]

## SUGAR'S EFFECTS ON THE BRAIN

There are many unhealthy foods available for purchase, but potato chips are particularly problematic. Scientists at the University of Erlangen found changes in more than eighty brain areas in lab animals after they consumed potato chips, especially in those areas that are connected to addiction, stress, sleep, attention, and gratification. Beyond that, the combination of carbohydrates and fat leads to gluttony (hyperphagia).[29] This and other studies support the theory that attention deficit hyperactivity disorder in children could be connected to an unhealthy diet, especially one with fast-food products that contain synthetic additives that affect the nervous system.

An important aspect to consider when thinking about the obesity epidemic is the wave of fat-reduced "light" products that flooded the market as a reaction to the generalized warnings against fat. Since reducing fat can lead to a loss in taste, manufacturers make up for this by adding more sugar, salt, or carbs to their "light" products. This creates new problems—mainly because consumers tuck in with great appetite because they believe that they can't gain weight from "light" products.

In the past, sugar was used sparingly as a spice and with a certain goal in mind—the dessert. In past centuries it provided only about three to four percent of nutritional energy. Today it's fifteen to eighteen percent. As we now know, sugar harms not only the teeth, but also the heart and the brain. Heightened blood sugar levels lead to decreased cognitive performance and ability to concentrate. Researchers such as the American biochemist Lewis C. Cantley believe that cancer is also caused by a high consumption of sugar.[30] It has already been established that overweight, diabetic people show a greater risk for cancer.[31]

Ultimately, sugar is mixed in with almost everything—pay attention to the fine print next time you go shopping. We find it in frozen pizzas, ketchup, yogurt, sausage, and almost every convenience product. With the aid of sugar (and salt) it's possible to cover up any boring or bad taste. But it's not only the tricks of the food industry that cause us to eat too much sugar—there's also the fact that sugar is addictive. Our brain derives its entire energy requirement solely from sugar, and since it was scarce in the past, the brain reacts strongly to it, with happiness among other things.

Sugar is most radically condemned by the Californian pediatrician and metabolism researcher Robert Lustig. He has shown that lab animals, once used to sugar, react with the same symptoms as if they were suffering from heroine withdrawal when sugar is removed from their diet.[32]

So what can you do to eat healthier? Eat, for example, whole-grain instead of white-flour products whenever possible. The taste of whole-grain products have improved significantly, and as with everything, it's just a matter of getting used to it. Cake, pizza, and pasta can all work well with whole-grain flour. And don't fall into the fruit sugar trap. Many products are now labeled "with natural sweeteners" or "only contains fruit sugar." Using the word "fruit" here is designed to make us believe that the content is healthy. But unfortunately, that is not the case. Fruit sugar boosts fat synthesis in the liver and barely contributes to any feeling of satiety.[33, 34] For years, fruit sugar, aka fructose, was recommended to diabetics, because it causes no release of insulin. But, in turn, there is not a feeling of satiety in the brain—the hunger remains. A few years ago, the German Federal Institute for Risk Assessment advised diabetics to avoid foods sweetened with

fructose. By now we know that fructose heightens unhealthy cholesterol levels and causes fatty livers. In fruit, fructose is not that big of a
problem because fibers, nutrients, vitamins, and phytochemicals ensure a healthy balance. Honey contains fructose, too, but also many
valuable ingredients beyond that.

What's particularly bad is high fructose corn syrup, which is often
used in industrial food production because it is nonperishable and
cheap. It's suspected to be a risk factor for many illnesses.[35]

If you want to avoid fructose, you shouldn't consume too much
agave syrup, which is advertised as an alternative sweetener in organic
supermarkets. Agave syrup actually contains a lot of fructose—and so
does dried fruit. Today, a lot of people suffer from fructose intolerance, or more precisely, from fructose malabsorption.[36] Our bodies
are no longer able to sufficiently digest the amount of fruit sugar we
consume. The consequence is that without it having been digested, the
fruit sugar reaches the small intestine and large intestine, where bacteria begin to ferment it. Decomposition gases are thus formed, which
causes diarrhea, flatulence, and pain.

## A THIRD OF THE GLOBAL POPULATION
## IS SENSITIVE TO SALT

Another component that is often hidden in food is salt. Roughly a
third of the global population is sensitive to salt—which means that
they react to salt with an increase in blood pressure.[37] Still, that doesn't
mean that we should automatically recommend reducing salt to people
with hypertension. I advise my patients to perform a self-experiment
over the course of four weeks: Hardly use any salt and eat as little
bread as possible. If they can observe blood pressure clearly decreasing
in that period of time, then they have a salt sensitivity. Bread is one of

the major sources of salt. During such a self-experiment, you should also stay away from frozen and other convenience foods that have a high salt content. There is also a lot of salt in sausage (even more so in organic sausage, because it lacks other preservatives) and in cheese. For years, physicians and other scientists have been trying to get the food industry to reduce the content of salt, fat, and sugar in their products. But since there is a lot of money to be made from them, this effort has not yet come to fruition.

That some people react sensitively to salt is probably due to the fact that the buffering capacity of the kidneys, where sodium is egested, is overextended. Looking at evolutionary history, it makes sense that the body has the ability to retain salt, since natural foods are low in salt. With the beginning of preservation, such as pickling, the daily consumption of salt has increased from 0.04 ounces to 0.4 ounces—and that's where the problem begins.[38] Salt is contained in almost all ready-made foods, even in cookies. If you try cooking without salt for a while and substitute it with many delicious spices, you'll find that you hardly need any of it.

## GLUTEN: A MARKETING PLOY?

Whole wheat grain? Some are going to be taken aback by this recommendation of mine and ask about gluten. Gluten is a "glue" protein that causes the excellent baking characteristics of wheat. All other cereal flours produce bread with a smaller volume and a less elastic interior, which is why they are less popular. The "glue" proteins found in wheat consist of hundreds of protein components, among them gluten. It is imagined that during the Neolithic revolution about ten thousand years ago, when wheat entered the human diet, the immune system was faced with the challenge of developing an immune tolerance to the hitherto only very seldomly consumed gluten. So, the fact that most of us are able to process gluten is a very recent quality when we consider the whole of evolutionary history—and it can quickly be lost again, as a result of an intestinal infection for example.[39, 40]

Right now, the rows and rows of gluten-free products available in supermarkets are growing steadily, and these products are usually expensive. And so, naturally, everybody is talking about wheat. But it's a complicated matter, because we have to differentiate between three distinct disorders. The best-known and most severe disorder is celiac disease (formerly called sprue). This is an autoimmune disorder that can be assumed from the presence of specific blood values and genetic diagnostics and the diagnosis can then be verified by means of a gastroscopy. This disease actually does make it necessary to avoid gluten throughout one's lifetime. This means staying away from wheat, rye, and barley. About 0.71 percent of the population (1 in 141) in the United States suffers from celiac disease.[41]

Next, there is wheat allergy, which occurs quite rarely—the characteristic IgE-immunoglobulins can be traced in the blood of about 0.1 to 4 percent of the population. In 10 percent of millers, bakers, and pastry chefs, such an allergy develops as a consequence of the flour that is inhaled and which can lead to skin rashes and asthma.[42] Here, it's only wheat that needs to be avoided completely.

The third disease that exists is a sensitivity with a more complicated name—non-celiac gluten sensitivity (NCGS). This is what is commonly known as "gluten intolerance." An increasing number of people seem to be afflicted by it—estimates range from 0.6 to 6 percent—but at the same time, it's not certain whether this syndrome has anything to do with grains at all.[43]

In the United States, the number of people who avoid gluten has grown massively in the past couple of years, but no tests are able to provide physiological reasons for this development. Professional athletes state that they are able to perform better when their diet is gluten- or wheat-free. Popular books, such as *Wheat Belly* by the American cardiologist William Davis, claim that wheat is to blame for the increasing number of obese people. Davis in particular holds club wheat (Triticum compactum), which is widely cultivated nowadays, responsible for that. But there is no sufficient scientific proof for this claim and it seems a bit too simple for my liking. The gluten-free diet is just big business.

Physiologically speaking, it's unclear what non-celiac gluten sensitivity is and what causes it. You could put it like this: This syndrome is always present when people avoid wheat because of health problems. This can but doesn't necessarily have to be connected to gluten. Just like a positive outlook supports self-healing powers, the worry that something might be indigestible to us can cause health problems. This would be the placebo's counterpart, a "nocebo."

And yet this gluten sensitivity, or wheat intolerance, whatever you would like to call it, exists—especially in people suffering from irritable bowel syndrome. By now, the culprits of this disease are assumed to lie in certain proteins contained in wheat, the amylase and trypsin inhibitors (ATI) that are predominately found in newer types of wheat like club wheat. They protect plants from pest damage, but they can also have a negative effect on the immune system. If you suffer from irritable bowel syndrome, it might be worthwhile to try and adopt a gluten-free diet. In a study, patients with this disease were offered gluten-free or glutenous muffins without knowing which kind it was they were eating. Results showed that 70 percent of the patients who ate the muffins containing gluten encountered health problems, while only 40 percent of the patients who ate the gluten-free muffins encountered health problems.[44]

It's important to diagnose celiac disease unambiguously and to isolate it from other symptoms. In patients with celiac disease, as little as 100 milligrams of gluten a day can cause an inflammation of the bowels—that's three crumbs of bread. The tolerable amount is higher in people suffering from wheat intolerance. The wide choice of gluten-free products is a good thing for people afflicted with celiac disease, but I advise people with gluten intolerance to keep trying gluten and wheat every once in a while, in the form of whole-grain and organic products, and then observe their reaction. In our clinic, we learned that the Ayurvedic diet, for example, which contains hardly any bread or pasta, is able to help with this problem without people having to spend too much money on special foods.

## INTESTINAL BACTERIA: A WORLD FULL OF MYSTERY

Whether we are healthy or sick crucially depends on the microbiota, i.e., the cosmos of bacteria in our gut. The intestine is—in its capacity as a huge contact area with food, i.e., with the outside world—the place where the immune system is influenced to a great extent and where it's decided whether autoimmune diseases, possibly even cancer and arteriosclerosis, develop. By now, it is well known that the microbiota plays a decisive role not only in many rheumatoid diseases, in arthritis, allergies, Crohn's disease, and ulcerative colitis, but also in many neurological diseases like multiple sclerosis and Parkinson's—though we cannot yet say which therapeutic consequences can be drawn from this knowledge.[45]

I do hope this knowledge will lead to nutrition receiving more attention from the medical community than it has so far. What we eat can influence the composition of the intestinal bacteria and their many different strands. Yet another reason to follow a vegetarian diet is that health-promoting intestinal bacteria feed mainly on fibers—that's why they are called prebiotics. A study published in *Nature* showed that massive changes in the microbiota can be detected as soon as three to four days after a transition from an omnivorous diet to a plant-based diet. And when the matrix of the genes is sequenced, an anti-inflammatory effect can be observed immediately.[46]

It's already possible to describe individual interdependencies rather well: The consumption of lecithin—a fat-like substance that is found in egg yolks, meat, and, to a lesser extent, in soy—causes the microbiota in the bowel to produce a metabolic factor that fosters atherosclerosis quite powerfully. If you kill the microbiota by using antibiotics, this factor disappears from the body—this is an instance where the role of the bacteria can be noticed very clearly.[47]

A positive example for this is beets, which naturally contain more than 1,000 milligrams of nitrate per kilogram. When we eat beets, this nitrate is concentrated in the salivary glands and then transformed into nitrite by the bacteria in the mouth. The nitrite is then swallowed and turned into nitric oxide, a substance that protects the vessels in the gastrointestinal tract. It is this cycle that makes beets so healthy—with the aid of the bacteria. Not only does beet juice lower blood pressure, but if you drink about 0.26 or 0.53 quarts of it a day, it is almost like natural doping: Several studies have shown that drinking beet juice improves athletic performance.[48] Because of its vasodilating capacity beet juice is now even recommended to patients with congestive heart failure by cardiologists: It lowers the cardiac work.[49]

The crux, then, lies in the detail: Up until a few years ago, nitrate and nitrite were branded as undesirable components in food, because in conjunction with certain proteins they are carcinogenic. But there are subtle, yet important differences: If you consume nitrate in the form of meat, carcinogenic nitrosamine forms due to the amines also contained in meat. The nitrate contained in beet, however, doesn't link to the protein. The advantages of consuming vegetables rich in nitrate strongly outweigh the disadvantages.

**PATIENT HISTORY**

## Parkinson's Disease
*Ayurveda—Eating to Fight Tremors*

The patient was 44 years old, of sturdy build, and was the father of three children. He had always eaten a "hearty" diet—until he was diagnosed with Parkinson's (at quite a young age for this disease).

Parkinson's causes the brain's nerve cells to degenerate. Symptoms consist of shaking as well as other movement disorders. The patient suddenly lost the ability to fully stretch out his arm. His left hand shook when he tried to hold it still. He was able to work, but for how much longer?

People suffering from Parkinson's deteriorate slowly. There is no cure for this disease, not even in naturopathy. The progress of the disease can, however, be slowed down with medication. And it's possible to support the process of delay quite efficiently—especially with Ayurveda. This traditional Indian medicine achieves astonishing successes, particularly where neurological diseases are concerned.

Ayurveda distinguishes three constitutional types, the doshas. According to Ayurveda, the patient's disease was connected to a surplus of vata, so he was recommended a diet that would alleviate this "windy" side of him, which was putting a strain on the nerves. In his case this meant eating grounding vegetables such as pumpkin, turnips, or potatoes; meals ideally with liquid or sauce-like consistency; curries rather than dry vegetables. To meet the requirements of kapha, his fundamental constitution, he was advised to season everything well, to make his meals slightly spicy, and not to let his portions become too large. Today, the patient has eliminated most animal products from his diet—instead, he eats healthy foods such as legumes, seeds, nuts, broccoli, or sprouts.

The second therapeutic approach may sound repulsive to many, but it helps: oily enemas. They channel harmful substances from the intestinal mucosa. Followers of Ayurveda believe that the end of the large intestine is the main seat of vata. Enemas have a localized unburdening function, but they also change the milieu of the entire intestine and thus the nervous system.

The patient also practices yoga, because the slow breathing soothes. Once a week, he undergoes an Ayurvedic oil massage that relaxes body and soul. He's been able to continue his work as a freelance caterer, but he has reduced the number of jobs he takes.

## MILK: NOT A HEALTHY FOOD

Metabolic processes in our bodies take place in a watery environment. The high number of enzymatic and other chemical processes demand a constant pH value, one that varies within a slightly alkaline range (between 7.35 and 7.4) as a standard value in the body. Even slight deviations from this are irreconcilable with being alive. In an intensive care unit, doctors work with a machine that measures the arterial-blood gas. Whether patients are approaching death can be detected, among other indicators, by the fact that the blood becomes acidic, that acidosis (acute overacidification) sets in.

But it's not like pH value is the same all over the body. In the stomach, for example, it's quite acidic—between 1.2 and 1.3. Bile is alkaline, measuring 7.4 to 7.7. Saliva has a value of 6.8. The feces should have a pH value somewhere between 6 and 7.

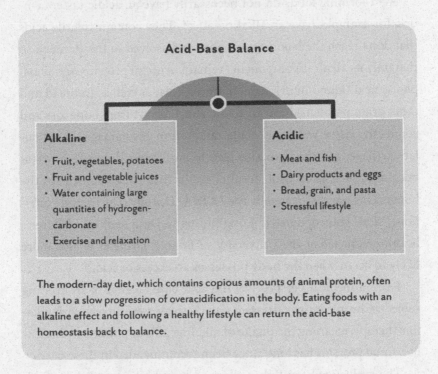

**Acid-Base Balance**

**Alkaline**
- Fruit, vegetables, potatoes
- Fruit and vegetable juices
- Water containing large quantities of hydrogen-carbonate
- Exercise and relaxation

**Acidic**
- Meat and fish
- Dairy products and eggs
- Bread, grain, and pasta
- Stressful lifestyle

The modern-day diet, which contains copious amounts of animal protein, often leads to a slow progression of overacidification in the body. Eating foods with an alkaline effect and following a healthy lifestyle can return the acid-base homeostasis back to balance.

Regulation of the acid-base balance is achieved by an elaborate buffer system. The two most important organs in this process are the lungs, which exhale carbon dioxide, and the kidneys, which expel bicarbonate and thus regulate pH value. This system is highly efficient. But when it is overworked, the body mobilizes minerals that are removed from the bones—which leads to osteoporosis. A second mechanism takes place in the connective tissue, which dries out as a result and becomes sensitive to pain. An excess of acid in the body becomes increasingly problematic as we age, because as functionality of the kidneys decreases so does the general buffer capacity. When other factors such as chronic inflammation are added to that, and if acid-forming foods make up the majority of a person's diet, health likely suffers.

Acid-forming foods do not necessarily have an acidic taste. Lemons, for example, have an alkaline effect. They contain volatile acids that don't reach the bloodstream but are dissolved in the stomach so that only its alkaline components remain. Animal proteins and phosphoric acid (found in drinks containing cola, as well as in bread and other grain products) have an acidic effect. Apart from bone loss and connective tissue weakness, acids can presumably damage the articular cartilage, and they can also lead to an increased release of stress hormones such as cortisol, another factor that causes damage to the bones. This was discovered by the DONALD study (Dortmund Nutritional and Anthropometric Longitudinally Designed) on children's health conducted at the University of Bonn.[50] Diabetes is also more likely to occur when the body possesses an excess of acid.[51]

From a medical perspective, the acid-base balance is an exciting subject: Chronic kidney diseases can be treated effectively with alkaline therapy, meaning the intake of alkaline pills or powder. A diet low in animal proteins has long since been recommended in these cases.[52]

The evaluation of milk has changed completely due to these findings. For a long time, it was thought that the calcium it contains protects the bones. Today we know that it's the other way around: Due to the acidity that milk produces in the body, the discharge of calcium far exceeds the calcium we ingest. Dairy products actually produce a negative calcium balance and are not a treatment method for osteoporosis.[53]

It is not possible to describe how much acid certain foods produce with complete accuracy. But there are the so-called PRAL values (Potential Renal Acid Load)—a formula influenced by acid-promoting factors like the sulfurous amino acid and phosphoric acid as well as protective factors (minerals, potassium, or calcium). They have been developed by the nutritionists Thomas Remer and Friedrich Manz and provide good points of reference.[54] They show that meat, cheese, some nuts, every type of grain, and even fish (especially if it's tinned, with tuna at the head of the pack) are acidic. My personal surprise was that black espresso, which I love, isn't acidic, but slightly alkaline.

All of this demonstrates, once again, the advantages of having a plant-based diet, avoiding meat and fish, and consuming only small amounts of cheese. If you do actually want to "cheat" every once in a while, it helps to drink a glass of orange or vegetable juice along with your meal. That buffers the acidity and ensures a healthy balance. Mineral waters rich in bicarbonate (also called hydrogencarbonate) are also useful, especially if you suffer from a chronic disease. You can also take Bullrich salt or alkaline powder—these are often administered in detox clinics. The studies invoked as evidence for this, however, have no actual quality. I stick to my belief that it makes no sense to have a bad diet and then take pills to counteract it.

There are commercial alkaline fasts which involve eating potatoes and root vegetables, i.e., a vegan diet rich in vegetables. In theory, this is certainly healthy, but it does not need the garnish sometimes added to it, things like tissue salts. Furthermore, alkaline fasting should not be confused with therapeutic fasting, which achieves a much stronger effect.

If you wish to do more about overacidification in your body, you should try "pranayama," yogic breathing exercises in which more acid is exhaled. Sweating in a sauna also relieves the body.

## LA GRANDE BOUFFE: THE BIG FEAST

"Having lost sight of our objectives, we redoubled our efforts." This quote by Mark Twain pops into my mind whenever I read studies on nutrition, nutritional deficiency, and obesity, such as the study on the effects on the metabolism of a "big feast" conducted by the research team headed by Guenther Boden.[55] The researchers gave volunteers 6,000 kcal of an unhealthy "Western" diet every day for a week. This is almost three times more than is recommended for daily consumption. But if you have ever traveled on a cruise ship and seen the buffets and all-you-can-eat specials, you know that such an extensive intake of food can happen in everyday life.

In the study carried out by Boden and his team—which insiders call the AIDA study—the excessive eating had lasting effects on the participants' health. On average, they gained about 7.7 pounds in weight, and the first stage of a diabetes mellitus was already looming. This was attributed to the oxidative stress (harmful free radicals) that was triggered by the excessive intake of calories. So far, it all makes sense. However, the researchers arrived at a strange conclusion. From the realization that excessive food has devastating consequences for healthy men even after just a few days, the following conclusion was drawn: ". . . our results (demonstrate) the urgent necessity to develop medications that reduce the oxidative stress." The scientists did not draw the obvious deduction that the results show how important it is to have a healthy diet that is low in calories.

After all, the opposite is possible, too: In two studies, a research team headed by Sarah Steven showed that diabetes mellitus is even curable by an eight-week fasting period.[56] This possibility had been completely ruled out by internists and diabetologists up until a few years ago. It was presumed that the pancreas was exhausted forever and would never again be able to produce insulin.

# Diabetes
## *Taming Hunger*

The architectural draftsman was 5'4" and weighed 220 lbs.—
obesity is not rare in our patients. Often, this obesity stems from a
medical therapy which, unfortunately, has become the norm: insulin. Almost ten percent of the population suffers from pancreatic
exhaustion, i.e., type 2 diabetes. Since the body is unable to produce sufficient amounts of insulin, this growth-inducing hormone
is replaced by medication.

In practice, this leads to a negative spiral: The patients gain
weight, move less and less, and the changed metabolism causes
cells to become resistant against insulin. This, in turn, heightens
blood sugar levels and as a consequence the patients receive even
more insulin. This creates the vicious cycle that led this patient,
who had been suffering from diabetes for twenty years, to weigh-
ing 220 lbs.—thus increasing her risk for atherosclerosis and cardiovascular diseases. The fact that she had also been diagnosed
with rheumatism, and cortisone therapy had become necessary in
the interim, put an additional strain on her insulin balance—it fluc-
tuated so heavily that she had to eat a snack at three in the morning
so as not to become hypoglycemic.

The patient, by now in her mid-sixties, learned to practice fasting, which significantly reduced her need for insulin. When she
came to our clinic, she needed 102 units of insulin daily. When she left
it was down to fifteen. Thanks to fasting and treatments in a cold
chamber, her rheumatic pains also improved. The swelling in her

wrists and ankles went down, the patient has lost 22 lbs., and she
is now much more agile.

What stopped this negative spiral? Fasting. It is like a reset button: The sugar-insulin system is interrupted. When the body is in a
constant state of hunger for a week, the cells activate new receptors through which they can channel in sugar—after all, they aim to
utilize everything they can get in times of need. When the patient
starts eating again after a fasting cure, the sugar can get to the cells
more easily thanks to the new receptors—and the body needs less
insulin.[57] Coldness is an additional stimulus that increases sensitivity to insulin. In type 1 diabetes, the stage in which the pancreas is
no longer able to produce insulin, the hormone has to be substituted. Type 2 diabetes, however, the much more common disease,
can be effectively treated with lifestyle therapies.

The architectural draftsman kept up a 1,400-calorie diet for
two weeks after fasting to maintain a low insulin level. It wasn't
hard, because her body was no longer urging her to eat constantly.

## THE VEGETARIAN LIFESTYLE

Ten more healthy years—that's the promise made by a diet and lifestyle
that has been studied by Seventh-day Adventists in Loma Linda, California, for years. This religious community treats their bodies like
temples.[58] They reject alcohol and nicotine and are completely devoted
to a healthy life. They go for frequent walks and cultivate close social
networks. For these reasons, Loma Linda is one of the "Blue Zones," in
which the most healthy, old-age people live. For some of the Seventh-
day Adventists, the vegetarian diet is an essential part of this recipe for
success. The vegetarians among the Seventh-day Adventists suffer

fewer heart attacks and strokes, and show fewer cases of intestinal cancer and diabetes compared to non-vegetarians within the community.[59]

Time and again, it has become clear that Asian and Mediterranean diets are healthier than Western diets. The reason for this is that they contain far fewer animal proteins or even avoid them completely. This raises the question: Why do we eat meat if it is killing us? Wouldn't it make sense for us all to become vegetarian?

In discussions on the issue of vegetarianism, I am frequently faced with this argument: Over the course of evolution humans have long been omnivores, which is why a purely plant-based diet must be nonsense. Fair enough, I answer then, but the situation has changed by now. We no longer wander for forty to fifty miles a day like the hunters of the Masai. Following a Stone Age diet (the Paleo diet) with large quantities of meat while living with central heating and driving around in our cars doesn't go well together.

Michael Greger, an American physician and best-selling author, is an active spokesperson for the vegetarian diet. He is critical of the fact that the negative effects of animal proteins have been made light of by nutritionists for decades while proteins of vegetable origin were denigrated. Greger calls this the "Great Protein Fiasco." It led to the vegetarian diet being judged negatively because it was believed that plants didn't contain enough proteins. At the same time, recommendations for protein intake were constantly revised upward even though there was no scientific evidence to substantiate these alterations.

It might have helped to take a look at breast milk. We can safely assume that evolution "designed" breast milk in such a way that it offers the biggest possible benefit for the child. It's striking here that breast milk shows a low protein content.[60] That is also one of the reasons why it can actually be risky to give infants cow's milk. And ultimately, it is an indication that we need far less protein than we assumed thus far.

Over the past few years more and more studies have proved how unambiguously animal protein heightens the risk of cardiovascular diseases, strokes, and diabetes.[61] So far, it has not been possible to fully explain why this is so. Supposedly, there is a connection there to the already-mentioned sulfurous amino acids that are the building blocks of proteins. They cause inflammatory processes in the body. In animal proteins their share is larger than in vegetable proteins.[62]

In a Harvard study, the effect of animal and vegetable proteins was compared in 130,000 test subjects. On average, their diet contained 14 percent animal proteins and 4 percent plant-based proteins. When the subjects were divided according to the frequency of their consumption of animal proteins versus vegetable proteins, strikingly clear health differences became apparent over the years. The consumption of predominantly vegetable proteins, the researchers found, was connected to significantly lower mortality from cardiovascular diseases. As a result, the researchers worked out the following formula: If a mere 3 to 14 percent of animal proteins is replaced by vegetable proteins, the risk of an early death is lowered considerably. This effect is particularly noticeable when sausage and otherwise highly-processed red meat is substituted by plant-based proteins—minus 34 percent. In second place follows the benefit of avoiding eggs—minus 19 percent. The exchange of non-processed red meat for plant-based proteins still adds up to a 12 percent lesser risk. Animal protein has a particularly severe effect on the risk of developing diabetes.[63]

Some nutritionists and physicians object to a diet low in meat and milk, arguing it would lead to muscle loss and osteoporosis. But that is wrong. A large-scale Swedish study demonstrated that the risk of developing osteoporosis actually increases if multiple glasses of milk are drunk every day.[64] Scientists at Harvard University, who were also researching the consumption of milk in children and adolescents, found no benefit but, instead, disadvantageous tendencies. In this long-term study, they assessed, among other issues, the frequency of femoral neck fractures decades later, during adulthood. The calcium in the milk offered absolutely no protective effect. On the contrary, in men who were drinking a lot of milk, the rate of fractures was even a little higher than in the average of the male population. On average, they were also taller, which heightened their risk. The fact that milk also contains growth hormones is well known.[65]

The consumption of meat also causes stress hormone levels to rise. A single meal containing meat is enough for this to happen. If consumers undergo a stress test after eating meat, they have been shown to be less stress-resistant than people who ate a purely plant-based meal. Since stress is linked to cancer risk, all of this likely contributes to the fact that animal protein promotes cancer.[66]

So what conclusions can we draw? Should we all become vegetarians? If you take everything we've discussed into consideration along with the myriad issues tied to industrial livestock production—the ethical problems, the environmental damage, and the energy requirements—it seems difficult to disagree with the merits of following a vegetarian lifestyle.

## VEGETARIAN OR VEGAN?

Even so, many people find it difficult to imagine life as a vegetarian. Presently, German men eat an average of 41.6 oz (2.6 lbs) of meat a week and women eat 21 to 24.7 oz. In the United States, the numbers are even worse: The average American now eats roughly 193 pounds of beef, pork, and/or chicken a year (or more than 3.7 pounds a week), up from roughly 184 pounds in 2012.[67, 68] The German Association for Nutrition still considers—strangely enough—10.6 to 21 oz to be reasonable, even though meat has almost no nutritional value, as you are about to see, but contains many risk factors: saturated fats, animal proteins, antibiotic residue, hormones, viruses, and persistent organic pollutants (suspected to be the causal agents of weight gain). Beyond that, unhealthy polycyclic aromatic hydrocarbons are produced during grilling, frying, and smoking.

By choosing to eat less meat you enter a simple exchange: The less meat you eat, the more you eat of other things. If these other things are healthy vegetables, whole grains, legumes, and nuts, you greatly lower your risk for chronic diseases. All the vitamins and phytochemicals these foods contain prevent cancer, arteriosclerosis, hypertension, bacteria, viruses, free radicals, and inflammations.

But naturopathy isn't ever prone to formulating universal rules—its focus is always on individual tolerability. The nutritionist Franz Xaver Mayr was the first to observe that a diet of raw food, healthy as it may be, doesn't agree with everybody.[69] As the German proverb goes: "What agrees with the blacksmith, makes the tailor sick"—it may be an old saying, but it still holds true. Someone who is very physically active will be able to eat more raw foods, more "cold" meals. Less physically active people should steam their meals lightly according to the Asian/Ayurvedic tradition or season their food accordingly (cabbage salad with plenty of caraway seeds, for example).

But that said, I no longer ascribe as much importance to individual tolerability as I did ten years ago. Research on the microbiome has shown that the body is able to adapt to a change in dietary habits rather quickly, within days or weeks. Still, attentiveness doesn't go amiss: In winter, the body has a demand for root vegetables, cabbage, or legumes rather than zucchini, strawberries, or watermelon. In summer, cinnamon, a warming spice, has no place in our food. And it's important to take the time to chew slowly. You also shouldn't drink anything while you eat so as not to dilute the digestive juices with additional liquid.

In the past, my favorite dish was roast pork with spaetzle. But I

realized that one's tastes change after a few weeks of following a vegetarian diet. Suddenly you enjoy vegetables, legumes, fruit, berries,
and nuts because of the multitude of their flavors. You'll also notice
that your general well-being increases quite quickly. Initial studies
have shown that the transition to a vegetarian diet is accompanied by
an improvement of the general mood.[70] The comparatively bad mood
of meat eaters is possibly caused by the metabolic products developed
by animals kept in factory farms up until their transport and slaughter.

There was an exciting experiment organized by ZDF, a German
television network: Volunteers were provided with vegan meals for
several weeks. A second group received dishes that contained meat. In
both cases, the meals were excellent: The first group was catered for by
the renowned vegan chef Attila Hildmann, the second was cooked for
by the no-less-famous chef Alfons Schuhbeck. I was tasked with su-
pervising both groups medically. Of course, no scientific conclusions
can be drawn within the framework of such an experiment. But I noticed that the participants who were eating vegan food seemed to be in
a much better mental state.

Lacto-vegetarian with small amounts of organic dairy products is
an excellent, healthy diet. Vegan isn't necessarily healthier, but for
some it's the preferred choice, mainly for ethical reasons. However, the
transition to a vegan diet poses a challenge. I advise my patients to try
a lacto-vegetarian diet, since cheese, yogurt, and other dairy products
do indeed widen the spectrum of available foodstuffs considerably.
When eating milk and cheese, try and eat wholesome organic products if possible. If a vegan diet is a viable option for you, pay attention
to a diverse choice of vegetables, nuts, and whole-grain products as
well as a sufficient supply of vegetable protein. Legumes and whole
wheat products contain a lot of plant-based protein, which should be
eaten in sufficient amounts particularly by people over the age of sixty,
when the demand for protein increases. For vegans it's important to

substitute vitamin B12, because a lack of B12 can lead to serious neurological diseases or dyscrasia. A very good way, apart from taking vitamin B12 drops, is using toothpaste containing B12.

## EGGS ARE NOT HEALTHY

I'm often asked how healthy eggs are. Study results have indicated that diabetics who eat eggs show a heightened risk for heart disease and strokes.[71] A study that was published in the *New England Journal of Medicine* in 2013 also showed that lecithin, found in high concentration in egg yolk, is transformed into a risk product for cardiovascular diseases and diabetes via the metabolism of the gut bacteria.[72]

In addition, there is the fact that eggs are often polluted by germs and toxins, by salmonella and other pathogens. This has led me to advise my patients to avoid eating eggs. A weekly "cheat day" can help you in the early stages of the transition to cutting eggs out of your diet. On that cheat day, you can "sin." This helps prevent the desire you normally experience when forced to give up something.

Another question I get asked a lot is whether there is a point in buying meat substitute products. Organic supermarkets are full of soy schnitzel, seitan burgers, or tofu sausages. If it's hard to refrain from eating the meat version, these products may be a little prop. I, too, eat some of them occasionally. But ultimately, it's not only about omitting meat from your diet in the long run, but to eat vegetables and fruit instead of seitan or tofu.

However, a diet without animal products is not automatically healthy. Vegetarian or vegan food can also be quite unhealthy, if it consists mainly of pasta, desserts, and ready-made meals. This phenomenon is called "pudding vegetarianism." But if you have a diverse vegetarian or vegan diet (learning to cook is fun!), it is exceptionally healthy—so healthy, in fact, that one has to be careful when taking additional medication. This was pointed out by Kim A. Williams, former president of the American College of Cardiology, who has been adhering to a vegan diet since 2003. His own LDL cholesterol (Low Density Lipoprotein, aka, the "bad cholesterol") levels fell from 170 to 90 milligrams per deciliter. In the beginning, this can even cause hypoglycemia and circulation problems, because insulin levels drop significantly.[73] But you can be mindful of that.

The extent to which a vegan diet lowers the levels of LDL cholesterol in the blood is truly impressive. This was confirmed by another study from 2003 published in the American journal *JAMA*.[74] Unfortunately, since then the belief has prevailed that only lipid-lowering medications are potent enough to lower cholesterol levels sufficiently. These medications are not actually more effective than a vegan diet. In addition to lowering cholesterol levels, a vegan diet also reduces important inflammatory factors in the blood, which contribute to the occurrence of heart attacks.[75] Once again, this presents the opportunity to recommend a healthy diet instead of resorting to medication immediately.

It's a good thing that we have statins—they do help many people. But they have side effects; 10 percent of patients experience muscular pains because of them and are thus deterred from undergoing therapeutic exercise, which represents the second big pillar of heart therapy.[76] Additionally, people who take statins have a worse diet in the long run than they did before they took statins.[77] Medications like these influence the way we think: Oh well, it doesn't matter what I eat, after all, I'm taking the pills. I tell patients what the medical guidelines say and recommend that. But if they are reluctant to take even more medication (because for hypertension, diabetes, and heart diseases doctors often prescribe multiple pills to be taken simultaneously), and if they experience severe side effects, I suggest trying a vegan diet for a change.

In hotels I always pay attention to what guests put on their plates for breakfast. Usually it's scrambled eggs and sausages. When you're standing in front of an inviting buffet, start with the plant-based part—fruit or raw foods. Then you'll have satisfied the biggest hunger before you give in to temptation at the other end of the table.

Men are a special risk group. They often eat twice as much meat as women. The consumption of meat is even considered an attribute of masculinity. But actually, testosterone levels are lowered by meat consumption.[78] I myself have been eating lacto-vegetarian for ten years and my experience was similar to that of quitting smoking. The first three months were hard, and I had to rein myself in a couple of times when I saw something delicious in a restaurant. But after those three months I stopped craving meat and today I don't even like the smell of meat anymore. In my own family, I have observed that children become accustomed to a vegetarian diet easily.

## ORGANIC SAUSAGES ARE NOT THE ANSWER

A short while ago, I saw a father and his son shopping for what seemed to be a "boys' weekend" in an organic supermarket: Their shopping cart was filled with pretty much everything that is unhealthy—meat, sausages, chips, cookies filled with marzipan, frozen pizzas, and french fries—though it was all organic. But by no means does "organic" mean that the products are healthy, even though naturally produced meat may indeed be of higher quality than meat produced in a factory farm—and thus has fewer harmful consequences.

Even though Germans love meat, they place—with the exception of the example I just mentioned—no great value on quality. In surveys, large parts of the population state that they oppose industrial livestock production and would be willing to spend more money on high-quality meat. However, this attitude is not reflected in reality. You could say, the spirit is willing, but the flesh is ... well, you know. Most populations in the Western world, with the exception of Mediterranean countries, spend very little money on food, only 10 percent of the per capita income. They are, however, strident in demanding more animal protection. And yet they buy cheap meat. Bigger and bigger animal factories are built in order to supply this demand. The argument for animal protection reinforces the case for a vegetarian diet.

For some time now, it's not only vegetarian food that has been trending, but vegan food in particular. A vegan or plant-based diet is, when done right and supplemented with vitamin B12, the healthiest form of nutrition according to current scientific knowledge.[79] Unfortunately, this realization is overpowered by ideological battles. "Vegan" is often used as a battle cry. Scientists like the cardiologist Kim A. Williams, whom I cited earlier, make themselves unpopular rather quickly when they add a vegan diet to the recommendations for their patients. When I visited Stanford in 2000, I asked a professor at the Preventive Medicine Research Institute to put me in touch with the physician and vegan Dean Ornish, who advocates changing your diet and lifestyle as a means to treat and prevent heart disease and who was and is a hero to me, to do a research project on heart health. This professor, however, just looked at me grimly and said, "We don't like him."

But dogmatism isn't getting us anywhere. Simply reciting studies and facts doesn't help most people change their lifestyle—we must build bridges to make these changes more accessible and attainable for all. Of course, wanting to make the entire population of America vegan is completely unrealistic. The philosopher and cultural scientist Harald Lemke, who worked a lot on the ethics of nutrition and gastrosophy, makes the case for moving toward a revolution in food culture using culinary curiosity rather than dogmatism: "What happens to a celery root when you vacuum-pack it or poach it at low temperatures?" he writes. "What do we have to do to shepherd's purse and bishop's weed in order to change the world? Those who know how to handle artichokes or sweet cicely don't need veal bones to get some zest into a stock."[80]

I would be glad if this has stirred up some of your own curiosity.

# CHAPTER SIX

# Stagnation Is Cause for Illness

## *The Importance of Exercise*

t took many decades for the entire medical world to come to the realization that physical activity stimulates important processes of protection, repair, and development in the body that have a health-promoting effect. Today, we know from scientific data that physical activity has proven itself to be an effective treatment in almost all illnesses. During my years of training as an internist, it was still standard for heart attack patients to remain in bed, more or less motionless, for three days or more. Today it's become clear that absolute bedrest is completely wrong and that rest in general is counterproductive in most illnesses.

In naturopathy, physical activity has always been among the most important therapies. Otto von Bismarck's recovery, aided by his personal doctor Ernst Schweninger, who was the head of the first naturopathic hospital in Berlin at the time, provides an early success story.

Germany's first chancellor was in frail health—plagued by rheumatism and diabetes, bad blood values and obesity, and on top of that, depression. The physicians at the Charité Hospital wanted to prescribe bedrest and a nourishing diet. Instead, Bismarck listened to Schweninger, who advised him to take daily walks and adhere to a low-calorie diet. Bismarck regained his health and to thank Schweninger, helped him gain a professorship at the Charité Hospital in 1884.[1]

## HOW MUCH PHYSICAL ACTIVITY IS IDEAL?

Naturally, in centuries past, the benefits of physical activity were not taken into consideration by conventional medicine because the ailment of our time, immobility, was rare back then. The working population moved a lot, because the level of motorization and automatization was still low. The majority of people were dealing with entirely different problems, such as, for example, infectious diseases. By now, though, there is an overwhelming number of studies that prove how important physical activity is, not only as a means of prevention, but also for treatment of diseases. Only in severe feverish conditions or ailments that are accompanied by great weakness is bedrest actually appropriate.

Other than that, the list of the diseases that can be positively influenced by physical activity is impressively long. It spans from cardiovascular afflictions—prevention of strokes and heart attacks, as well as the lowering of accompanying risk factors like diabetes, hypertension, obesity, and lipid metabolic disorders—to rheumatic diseases. In painful arthroses in particular, physical activity benefits the synovia and trains the supportive muscles. Likewise, in inflammatory rheumatic diseases like Bechterew syndrome, physical activity is the most important course of treatment since it helps maintain the flexibility of the spine. In osteoporosis, physical activity strengthens the microstructure of the bones through the accompanying vibrations.

Even depression is successfully treated with physical activity—in mild and intermediate cases it's as similarly effective as psychotropic drugs.[2] For cancer patients, physical activity is essential: Based on many studies, it's estimated (unfortunately, the range of assumptions is quite large) that about 15 to 25 percent of breast cancer cases can be avoided through regular physical activity.[3] For intestinal cancer, this figure is at 30 to 40 percent,[4] for aggressive types of prostate cancer it's 50 to 65 percent.[5] And finally, even pain diseases like migraines, neck or back pains, as well as fibromyalgia, can be contained successfully through physical activity.

Unfortunately, we have not succeeded in getting people moving thus far. In the 1970s, fitness trails were created in nature and since then there have been countless attempts to motivate the population to exercise and engage in more physical activity. The numbers were and are, however, depressing. Scientifically speaking, this is called kinesophobia—the fear of physical activity. This is not limited to the proverbial weaker self, the inability to motivate yourself to exercise. Many patients also experience pain when they move. During each of my rounds, I work at convincing them that movement is still good for them, even though they initially feel like they should rest instead.

How much physical activity is ideal? There are prudent guidelines that recommend three rounds of 45 minutes of aerobic exercise a week (135 minutes)—physical activity, that is, which is dosed in such a way that you don't even run out of breath. Some recommendations include, depending on the illness, five hours (300 minutes) a week, favoring almost double. All of this has been scientifically proven, but what use is it to us if those are completely unrealistic goals? Many naturopathic physicians, but also one of Germany's "popes of prevention," Martin Halle, professor at the Technical University of Munich, believe that we must lower the threshold for beginners in order to make the targets for physical activity achievable. And since many people have been traumatized by PE lessons in school, a moralistic appeal only accomplishes the opposite of the desired effect.

## FIND AN ACTIVITY YOU ENJOY

Ultimately, it's not all that important to measure "performance"—and counting calories when you are suffering from diabetes doesn't work either. The most important thing is to leave it up to you to take the initiative instead of fulfilling some kind of external goal. That's why you should choose a form of exercise that is fun for you. When I meet with patients who are limited in their ability to move, I ask them what sorts of things they enjoyed doing before. This is called *remembered wellness*. The memory of how you felt after a day of moving in the fresh air helps with motivation. Often, conversations like these lead to an impulse, an idea. Additionally, we always talk about what the patient's daily routine and the finances allow. Exercise has to bring joy, otherwise it is pointless.

Maybe the fact that you don't have to start a fitness training program takes away your fear of exercise. It's not necessary to go running; on the contrary, jogging or high-performance sports often lead to orthopedic problems. Marathon runners often suffer from gastric ulcers and a heightened level of atherosclerosis in the coronary vessels—this shows that their strain is too high, and the benefits of the exercise have turned into damage. That's why the so-called couch potatoes stand to gain the most: When they are able to motivate themselves to exercise a little, maybe thirty minutes once or twice a week, they profit from this enormously.

For people to find motivation, they need to see hope for improvement. We can provide them with that—it's not that hard. For example, every kind of everyday activity is useful, like going for walks, which is something that can't be praised enough. Walking upright is our natural form of movement, as it corresponds to our physical preconditions.

My most important recommendation is this: Use every opportunity you get to walk a few steps. Ignore elevators or escalators and use the stairs; ride your bicycle to work; don't wait for the bus at the stop, but walk the three stops for which you were going to take it. It takes a while to reprogram yourself—I know this from personal experience. Before, I was satisfied when I was able to snatch a good parking spot and drive right up to where I needed to go with my car. Today, I appreciate it when I have to walk three blocks to my destination. Because I know it's true: Every step counts.

On weekends or on other free days, you should plan for longer periods of physical activity at a time: Two hours are ideal, preferably outside. In Japan, there is a tradition of "forest bathing"—*Shinrin-yoku*—which is by now an integral part of preventative health care in Japan and South Korea. This is also where initial studies on the subject have been conducted. Qing Li, a medical doctor at Nippon Medical School in Tokyo and one of the world's experts in forest medicine and immunology, was able to prove that forest bathing stimulates the activity of natural killer cells and anticancer proteins, thus strengthening the immune system.[6] In South Korea, thirty-four more "healing forests" are being created in addition to the three existing ones.

When comparing walking in an urban environment to walking in a natural setting, i.e., in a forest or a park, we find that important physiological parameters that are under the influence of the autonomic nervous system—such as the heart, blood pressure, and heart rate variability—improve in nature. Tension, fatigue, and depressiveness decrease.[7]

The stimulating and invigorating effect of nature even applies in a clinical setting. Roger S. Ulrich, an architect who specializes in building hospitals at the Chalmers University of Technology in Sweden, has followed patients whose gallbladder had been removed for nine years, from 1972 to 1981. Those who lie in hospital rooms with a window overlooking trees had significantly shorter convalescing periods than those who stared at nothing but walls.[8]

Findings like these show our evolutionary past, our connection to nature. Being in contact with nature reduces stress and relaxes us, according to a study from 2015. In a meta-analysis, Diana Bowler, at the Senckenberg Biodiversity and Climate Research Centre in Frankfurt, summarized the findings of twenty-five studies on the experience of nature and health and found clear indications for a positive mental effect. Accordingly, we suffer when we are estranged from nature, consciously or unconsciously.[9] In the United States, the term "nature deficit disorder" was created to reflect the consequences of increasing urbanization. Cities cause stress: The physician Kristina Sundquist and her team at the University of Lund were able to demonstrate that the numbers for depression and even psychoses are on the rise in this setting.[10] In an environment close to nature, on the other hand, activity in the prefrontal cortex, which is responsible for judgment, contemplation, and worry, decreases—after as little as ninety minutes outside.[11] Studies have shown that people who make long visits to green spaces have lower rates of depression and high blood pressure. Even visiting outdoor green spaces for thirty minutes or more during the course of a week has clear beneficial health effects.[12] Simply looking at forest scenery on a plasma screen for ninety seconds activates brain centers for relaxation, compared to looking at urban scenery.[13] We are currently conducting a study with Stefan Brunnhuber, the Medical Director of the Diakonie Kliniken in Zschadrass near Leipzig, in which we are investigating whether it's possible to treat psychological diseases with daily, ninety-minute walks in nature. The study is called "A Walk in the Park."

Since roughly 5 percent of adults in Germany suffer from depression that requires treatment, such findings are not trivial. The way we treat our natural environment has consequences, and in any case, there need to be sufficient public green spaces available in cities. Nature offers pleasant sensory impressions, "soft fascinations"—the greenery, the movement of the clouds, or the sounds of water don't exert the brain and allow it to recover. In cities, however, the stimuli are complex and concentrated and require permanent attention. Interestingly, merely looking at images of nature leads to relaxation—even though forest wallpaper may be totally out of fashion. Maybe you're not a fan of the outdoors, but natural materials in your apartment, like coconut coir matting or wood, calm the senses. But nothing comes close to the effect of taking a walk in the woods. Considering all physiological parameters, walking in the woods is notably superior to walking in the city or in a gym.

## TAKE A PLAYFUL APPROACH TO WALKING

Walking through the landscape at leisure has always been a privilege of the elite. You'll see this in the philosophical schools of ancient Athens, of the Epicureans and the Stoics, where conversations were held while walking or sitting in the garden, but also in the Baroque period or the Renaissance. Great importance was placed on experiencing nature. In 2004, an American diabetes researcher named Neville Owen discovered that aimless strolling is superior to walking for a specific purpose.[14]

Therefore, you should take a playful approach to walking. Step counters may be of help as long as you don't let yourself be terrorized by them but merely use them as a guide instead. You'll soon find that the daily ten thousand steps that are considered to be beneficial to our health nowadays aren't so easy to achieve. Step counters—which have been integrated into many smartphones by now—could serve to provide a kind of biological feedback and remind us to go get some fresh air and take a walk around the block.

I'm far less convinced by running, as I mentioned earlier. Not only can it cause problems with ankle and knee joints, it's also not a form of exercise that brings many people joy or that can be done throughout your entire life. But continuity is essential. This is shown in the case of the previously mentioned "Blue Zones," where many people live to the age of one hundred: In Loma Linda, California, many of these people are Seventh-day Adventists who walk a lot and do so quite fast. Similarly, the people living on the Nicoya peninsula or the island of Sardinia move a lot while working as farmers or shepherds. Beyond the physical exercise, the vitamin D and daylight that come from being outside are additional health-promoting factors.

If you can manage to exercise intensively for 150 minutes a week, maybe even for 300 minutes, you'll be rewarded with an enormous benefit. Not only will you be preventing cardiovascular disease and diabetes, you'll also be reducing your risk of cancer, particularly your risk of breast or colon cancer.[15]

Furthermore, you maintain your weight by exercising. Patients often ask me why they gain weight as they get older even though they pay attention to what they eat. I then explain to them that they shouldn't move less, as is often the case, but on the contrary a little more each year. Since the metabolism reduces with age, the basal metabolic rate is lowered, as is the body temperature. That's why elderly people tend to feel cold more quickly. If you exercise, you build up your muscles at the same time. That also keeps you slim, because muscles require more energy than fat reserves. And for that matter, it also helps us feel warm.

On principle, I recommend three kinds of physical activity: endurance training, strength training, and coordination training. There is no need to go to great lengths for strength training, it's enough to place two dumbbells (5.5 or 10 lbs.) and a Thera-Band in locations you pass frequently and where you can do a few exercises here and there, but every day, of course. In addition, it's important to foster coordination, which decreases with age. That's the reason for the heightened risk for falls. Good exercises to help prevent this are walking backward in qigong, the one-leg stand in yoga, or using a small trampoline. I can wholeheartedly recommend qigong and tai chi in any case.

Overall, endurance sports are slightly superior to other forms of exercise, as they slow down the aging processes. A study conducted by cardiologists at the University Medical Center of the Saarland showed that the shortening of the chromosomes in cell division, which ultimately causes aging, is curbed by playing endurance sports.[16] But since there are additional risks that occur with age—as muscle deterioration leads to instability while standing or walking, for example—it's important not to neglect strength and coordination training over endurance training. Hop, jump, walk sideways or backward from time to time—variation is always good for you!

Interval training is also an interesting possibility. Physicians at the Saarland University in Homburg divided non-athletic, healthy volunteers aged thirty to sixty into different groups. Those who were asked to alternatingly sprint a short distance and then walk at leisure achieved results just as good as those who were going through continuous endurance training.

## TRAIN YOUR CONNECTIVE TISSUE

Physical activity also benefits the fasciae. These bands of connective tissue surround muscles and tendons and have been the focus of a new way of looking at the body. For a long time, the physician's gaze was focused on the skeleton. When the knee hurt, this was diagnosed as arthrosis caused by cartilage damage. If the back hurt, it was the spinal disk pressing on the nerves. Certainly, these phenomena can cause pain. But through recent clinical research it has become increasingly obvious that many of these diseases that cause pain have been successfully treated with therapies that don't change these signs of wear and tear yet still bring relief: massages, yoga, or acupuncture.

In these therapies, it's the connective tissue that has become the focus of attention. Modern imaging techniques allow for ever more delicate structures to be made visible. In the process, it became apparent that the connective tissue isn't just padding material in the body, but a highly active tissue that surrounds and connects all muscles and organs. There are the fascial tissues with tendinous properties, but also the more delicate intermediate layers that together form a full-body network. It ensures elasticity and slippage of muscles and organs as well as the joints surrounding them. If the fasciae lose their elasticity they become stiff or even inflamed, and numerous pain syndromes can develop as a result.

Furthermore, the fasciae are connected to pain trigger points. Many people with painful diseases know them, as they are points of maximal pressure pain. A good physical therapist can locate these pain trigger points accurately, and sometimes you can even find them yourself. These points, in turn, are connected to other remote areas, e.g., the foot fasciae that are interconnected up to the head. That's why a problem in the upper spine can have its actual causes in a heel spur, and vice versa.

The connective tissue possesses a great number of free nerves. This network of nerves enables proprioception, the perception of our position in space. It can also send out pain signals—studies with high-resolution ultrasound suggest that the flexibility of the different layers of connective tissue is often disrupted when that happens.[17] Experiments have shown that fasciae react to stress hormones such as adrenalin and noradrenalin. They contract and convulse—an indication that stress causes muscles as well as their essential elastic coating to harden.

The connective tissue nourishes the fasciae and in naturopathy it is assigned an important role in health maintenance. It swims in a matrix of sugar-protein compounds in which toxic substances or insufficiently developed proteins are disposed. Dehydration leads to withering and to a loss of the tissue's elasticity. Acidosis, which can be caused by wrong nutrition, e.g., by animal protein that acts as an acid in the tissue, can activate pain receptors and induce inflammation. When the fibroblasts, those cells in the connective tissue that produce the fiber structure of muscles and tendons, are overburdened as a result of dehydration or acidosis, the combination of overproduction and inflammation can result in tissue transformation and a painful fibrosis—a comparison that lends itself well here is that of a woolen sweater that was washed in water too hot.

This is exactly the point at which some naturopathic therapies start. By stretching the connective tissue with certain massage techniques, the healthy activity of the fibroblasts is stimulated. The same effect can be achieved with acupuncture—where the needle is placed and subsequently further stimulated by turning it. The meridian network of Traditional Chinese Medicine follows surprisingly close along broad bands of fasciae.

In 2009, I was rather astonished by one particular study. The discomfort of people suffering from carpal tunnel syndrome, a problem inside the hand, was significantly relieved if they received just a single cupping treatment in the neck area, in a completely different location from where the pain is felt, that is.[18] Today I know that the cupping probably stimulated the connective tissue and the fasciae fifteen inches removed from the area. That's also how we can explain the effect of the so-called foot reflex zones. It is considered disproven that the foot has reflex zones but massaging it can still have an effect on remote areas via the fasciae. In a similar way, the success of a *gua sha*, a Chinese scraping massage of the back to treat persistent neck pains, can be explained.

It is important to keep the connective tissue, which consists of up to 70 percent of water, moist. Presumably, physical activity and manual therapies mobilize and stimulate the water in the fasciae layer so that the entire area becomes supple again. Moreover, I am sure that nutrition plays a significant role in the elasticity of the connective tissue. During therapeutic fasting we can observe it recovering every single day—it's visible even to the naked eye. The tone of the underlying connective tissue and thus the tension of the skin improve, and often the dreaded cellulite disappears, not just through fasting, but just as much through a wholesome, vegetarian diet.

But what is the best way to keep the fasciae and the connective tissue in good working order? Yoga helps, because here the focus is on stretching. Cupping also creates pressure, as does the traditional deep tissue massage that reaches deep and may thus cause pain, but significantly improves a chronic pain condition after two or three treatments. A similarly positive effect is achieved by Rolfing—physical manipulation of the fasciae. Ida Rolf was an American biochemist who was propagating the fasciae's essential role as early as in the 1970s, at a time when their existence couldn't even be proven yet.

Special fasciae rollers and similar contraptions have been available for a few years now, but a spiky massage ball or stretches with short, bouncy, fast movements against the edge of the desk or the wall are adequate. This leads to microscopically minute tears in the tissue which initiate repair processes in the fibroblasts as a result. A well-dosed strain therefore benefits the fasciae, while an excessive strain causes them to wither—here, too, the principle of hormesis is at work.

## EXERCISES FOR PEOPLE WHO SIT A LOT

A few additional remarks on sitting: As a result of a daily routine that involves computers, smartphones, and tablets, people spend more and more hours every day sitting. Even the stroll to the wastebasket or to the colleague a few desks away has been made redundant by modern technology. The consequences of this are dramatic. Scientists are already speaking of the "sitting disease." Not only does sitting down for too long cause bad posture, accompanied by back and neck pain and headaches, it also increases the risk of developing diabetes by up to 90 percent, and the risk of cancer and heart diseases by 20 percent.[19] At least one hour of additional exercise a day is necessary to balance out the risk of an early death due to too much sitting.

But we shouldn't abstain from sitting down completely. We will always be sitting while driving a car and during meals. But it doesn't seem to be absolutely necessary to be sitting down all the time while working at a computer or during meetings. By now there are many suppliers of standing desks, and meetings can just as well happen while standing or walking—as part of a new work culture. Or as the poet Christian Morgenstern put it: "Thoughts—just like children and dogs—often want us to take them for a walk outside."

## Heart Disease
*Health Should Not Be Stressful!*

The healthiest life is useless if it stresses you out. I have learned this from two twin brothers who came to my office for a consultation. Both were, naturally, the same age, forty-six years old, but they were leading very different lives. One of them was a diplomat, always on the road with a driver, always ready to have a pleasant conversation. He was slightly overweight and had rosy cheeks. The other was a businessman who traveled a lot and owned houses in Sydney and London. Lean and fit, the tension he was under manifested itself in his face in the form of constant twitches. During a stay in Australia, the businessman had three stents put in place to keep his coronary vessels open after he had experienced a sudden feeling of faintness. Hearing this, his twin brother became worried—after all, he had the same genes.

The diplomat was in great health, even though he liked to drink good wine and eat fatty foods. On the other hand, after his heart trouble, the lean businessman followed every dietary recommendation he was able to find on the internet and exercised for precisely one hour every day. The first thing he did was ask me how many minutes exactly one was supposed to meditate, what available data there was, and also how many breaths he should take precisely in which yoga position. But he had not changed anything about the level of stress he faced at work.

Living healthfully with the sole aim of being efficient can have the reverse effect: If you can't relieve any pressure during exercise, if you are unable to relax even though you could benefit from a little rest, the stress hormones you accumulate can lead to inflammations in the cells of blood vessels. In the walls of the vessels, these often trigger the immune system's repair processes which then lead to undesired residue in the vessels and finally dangerous blood clots. What this businessman and his heart needed most of all was rest. But he had a very hard time getting it. Four months after our meeting he had an additional bypass surgery, after his heart's condition kept worsening. His diplomat brother, however, is doing great. He has his heart checked every few months, eats healthy but with pleasure, and doesn't allow himself to be tyrannized by health dogmas.

The example of these two brothers demonstrates that while it is good and right to strive for a healthy lifestyle, if this pursuit is turned into a high-performance life, it doesn't achieve anything. Of course, there are people who draw internal satisfaction from high performances, who can live well with constant stress. But most people don't admit to themselves that they are only giving it their all because in periods of calm they would find that they aren't happy with their life. Feeling happiness, no matter what life throws at you, is an important building block of health.

# CHAPTER SEVEN

# Yoga, Meditation, and Mindfulness

*Mind-Body Medicine*

S tress is the most severe risk factor for health in the twenty-first century. Even children are affected: In a 2015 study on stress, one in six children and one in five adolescents already showed clear symptoms of stress. In a survey carried out by the German medical insurance company Techniker Krankenkasse in 2016, 60 percent of the adults interviewed stated that they were agitated, and almost 25 percent declared that they were frequently under stress.

The most important stress factors are work (46 percent), high expectations of oneself (43 percent), a full schedule outside of work (33 percent), traffic (30 percent), as well as constant digital availability (28 percent). The stress level was especially high in those professionals (30 percent) who never turn off their smartphone, who are "always on," in other words.

Stress heightens the risk of heart attacks and strokes, tumors and immune diseases, depression, and much more. And it shortens your life. But as you might recall, I wrote earlier about how stress can also be healthy. Isn't there the positive eustress (controlled stress) and negative distress?

Over time, the scientific community has sometimes praised stress, other times it has been condemned completely in every shape and form. But the following viewpoint has finally emerged: Basically, four concurrent circumstances determine whether stress poses a healthy challenge or something that makes us sick. Those four factors are:

1. duration
2. intensity
3. how much control we can retain over it
4. whether the reasons for which we take on stress are meaningful to us or not

There are no hard and fast rules for these four factors, no data on the dosage like there is for medication. It always remains an individual question of how much stress can be endured. One person's breaking point might be a comfortable level of stress for another person. But for everyone, a lot of stress increases the danger of becoming sick. Those who work more than fifty-five hours a week, as meta-studies from 2015 have shown, have a 33 percent higher risk of suffering a stroke, and a 13 percent higher probability of developing heart disease.[1]

Yet it probably doesn't depend on the number of hours. Happiness researchers like the Swiss economist Mathias Binswanger (*Die Tretmühlen des Glücks*, "The Treadmills of Happiness") have pointed out that while the weekly hours of work have reduced massively, and domestic work has become less demanding due to machines and ready-made foods, our time budget for relaxation has not increased accordingly.

The reason: Our free time has become filled with ever more tasks and to-do lists. On top of that, work processes have become more condensed and fast-paced. Prime examples of this are hospitals. The number of patients admitted has been doubling or even tripling year after year. Yet the basic workload for hospital personnel has stayed the same for each patient or has grown considerably. Gone are the times when doctors or nurses could catch their breath over a cup of coffee and have a conversation with colleagues. Even though actual working hours have been reduced, stress has increased because tasks have to be completed in a more efficient manner.

## How Can I Recognize Stress? The Symptoms of Stress

### Body

- Cold hands
- Pain in the back and/or the neck
- Tension in the shoulders
- Indigestion
- Insomnia
- Tinnitus
- Digestive problems
- Restlessness
- Fatigue
- Irritated eyes

### Behavior

- Excessive consumption of: alcohol, cigarettes, coffee
- Uncontrolled eating (ravenous hunger)
- Grinding of teeth
- Inability to complete tasks

### Emotions

- Fear, feeling of emptiness, doubts
- Irritability, anger
- Hostility
- Feeling unhappy for no apparent reason
- Arrogance

### Mind

- Forgetfulness
- Trouble concentrating
- Declining creativity
- Loss of a sense of humor
- Problems with decision making

## A LACK OF SLEEP AS AN INDICATOR FOR STRESS

As a result of their everyday stress, about 15 to 20 percent of Americans suffer from sleep deprivation and insomnia.[2] I have experienced this firsthand. During the four years of my internistic-cardiological training I had to work rotating shifts under great stress and never really had any time to recover or get enough sleep. Promptly, I contracted chronic sinusitis. All natural remedies—from Scotch hose treatments, saunas, and medicinal herbs to sole inhalations and exercise—were ineffective. At some stage, I had a surgery to widen my sinus cavities, which the ear, nose, and throat specialist had recommended. But the symptoms remained. I was at a loss. Eight months later, my time at the ICU was over and I transferred to the cardiac catheterization and ultrasound lab, a less stressful job with regular hours. My body was able to rest and recover, and the chronic sinusitis was gone within four weeks.

Irregular and insufficient sleep can also cause weight gain. A lack of sleep furthers insulin resistance via the hormonal cycles. The cells are unable to absorb glucose properly, and this in turn leads to a ravenous appetite, increased food intake, and weight gain. In addition, the immune system is weakened. On the other hand, the opposite extreme is also problematic: People who sleep for a very long time, i.e., more than nine hours a night, often suffer from health problems. Their tiredness is possibly a sign of a depressive mood or exhaustion. Therefore, it is necessary to find the right balance based on the individual daily routine. Not everyone has the genetic properties that enable them to manage with only four to five hours of sleep a night like Napoleon. I would recommend observing yourself attentively to figure out how many hours of sleep you need to feel well-rested. This may change somewhat with the seasons or when you are on vacation. Ayurveda recommends going to bed as early as possible, at 10 p.m. at the latest. If that's not possible, a short siesta in the afternoon, or a powernap, can complete the need for sleep.

## CONSTANT AVAILABILITY IS HARMFUL TO YOUR HEALTH

Sleep is the most delicate sensor of stress. But ensuring that stress doesn't arise in the first place is becoming more and more difficult for all of us. In part, this is due to the fact that technology has made all of us available around the clock. Handling digital media is ultimately a big medical experiment, because it's still not clear how it affects our health.

What is certain, however, is that the frequent use of screens causes increasing difficulty falling asleep and interrupted sleep phases—and consequently sleep deprivation. Among the causes here are not only the focused attention and muscular tension in general, but specifically the blue light emitted by the screens: It suppresses the sleep hormone melatonin. Newer models have a night mode that subdues the blue light. To reduce blue light as much as possible, you should use this mode during the day as well—it can be adjusted manually.

The digital network controls us. Having grown accustomed to quick response times, we've become increasingly impatient. Being forced to wait in front of a computer heightens blood pressure immediately, quickens the pulse, and leads to the release of stress hormones. A similar effect can be observed—and this is an intriguing comparison—when watching horror movies.

Because time always seems to be running out, we try to do multiple things at once—multitasking. This works quite well in predominantly automatized activities such as walking and talking, or driving and thinking. It does not work, however, when we are performing two or more demanding tasks at the same time; the brain is then forced to constantly switch back and forth between different activities. Multi-tasking, therefore, is a "multiswitching," exhausting and damaging to the nerves. The psychologist Matthew Killingsworth and his colleagues developed an app for an interesting experiment to measure our psychological state in everyday life by using a smartphone. The participants of the experiment constantly registered what they were thinking and doing at any given time. The result was published in the professional journal *Science* in 2010. The title of the article, "A Wandering Mind Is an Unhappy Mind," summarizes the findings: Whenever our thoughts drift, when we think of something other than what we are doing at the time, i.e., when we are multitasking, our brain exerts itself tremendously. As a result, we can become depressed and anxious.[3]

Anxieties and depressions are among the most common diseases around the world. Genetic and social factors as well as individual experiences are considered instrumental in whether we develop a depression or anxiety disorder. But using computers also contributes to this. According to a Japanese study of 25,000 office workers, the frequency of depressions rises after five hours of daily computer use.[4] The constant interruption of our thoughts caused by working online has consequences: In one experiment, participants were asked to write a letter and check their email simultaneously—their ability to perform the first task was reduced by half.[5, 6]

We should, therefore, focus on what we're doing at any given moment. But this also implies an act of letting go of certain things, which is not always so easily done. A simple measure to prevent stress consists of not using the smartphone while performing other tasks. For example, 90 percent of users are looking at their phones even when talking to someone else.[7] We can observe a so-called "rule of three" here: When five or six people sit together, it's enough for three of them to be involved in a conversation attentively to give the other three a reason to quickly check their text messages or email.

## STRESS OCCURS WHEN WE HAVE NO CONTROL OVER THINGS

Stress is aggravated when we have no control over it or can't see the purpose of it. This, for example, is why young parents rarely suffer from burn-out—despite sleep deprivation and permanent multitasking. Their exertion is compensated by the love for their child, they understand the purpose and meaning of their exertion. Mere sense of duty or pressure, however, are more burdensome.

Firdaus Dhabhar, a psychiatrist at Stanford University, is a neuro-immunologist and cancer researcher. He is concerned with looking at stress in a more differentiated manner. He has, for example, been able to show how short-term stress strengthens the body's defenses because it causes an increase of white blood cells.[8] A vaccination has a stronger effect when the body is exerted beforehand, for example by pedaling hard on a stationary bicycle.[9] But maybe it's not stress itself at all, but the relaxation after the exertion that has a positive effect. The fact that regular meditation fortifies this effect, as demonstrated by the American brain researcher Richard Davidson, is indicative for this as well.[10]

Like everything in nature, stress has two sides. Challenges have always advanced evolution: When flies or mice are put under stress, they live longer.[11] Stress activates the brain. A research group at the University of Bochum was able to show that we retain memories better under slight stress. Cortisol, one of the stress hormones, activates those parts of the brain that are responsible for long-term memory.[12]

Artists, musicians, or competitive athletes have all reported how important a certain level of tension is. A legendary example for this is

Oliver Kahn, the former goalkeeper for FC Bayern Munich, who pushed himself to extraordinary performances by using aggression when he was under stress. A thrill can mean pleasure and fulfillment, otherwise there wouldn't be people who sacrifice so much time and money to expose themselves to dangers—when free-climbing or base jumping, "danger freaks" feel fantastic. But if stress endures and the body gets no opportunity to relax, it facilitates forgetfulness, causes the ability to concentrate to dwindle, and increases the risk of dementia.

Fear of stress can be worse than stress itself. In an American study, thirty thousand people were asked how much tension they experience on a daily basis, how they deal with it, and whether they believe that it's unhealthy. Eight years later, it became evident that among the people suffering from stress, 40 percent of those who believed that it was harmful died younger. The others, who didn't attach too much importance to it, showed the lowest mortality risk of all comparison groups.[13]

In an experiment, researchers at Yale University conducted simulated job interviews in which the "staff manager" (an actor) put the participants under a lot of stress. Before that, one group was shown a movie that addressed the bad, health-damaging effects of stress. The other group was shown a movie which explained that stress promoted attentiveness and performance ability. In the second group, significantly lower levels of stress hormones in the blood were measured.[14] So, it's not always stress that's unhealthy, but the belief that stress is unhealthy.

People who feel like they have control over their personal circumstances are less affected by stress. This is verified, among other studies, by the much-cited Interheart study, a large-scale experiment on the most important risk factors for heart attacks conducted in fifty-two countries in 2004: The risk for suffering a heart attack was shown to be increased by 30 percent in those participants who were under stress and had little or no control over it.[15] A similar result was achieved by a British study among thirty thousand of the country's civil servants.[16]

But it's not just attitude—physical bearing also plays a part. In 2016, biologist Shwetha Nair and coworkers from the University of Auckland were able to show that a person's sense of self-worth is diminished when they adopt a slumped posture for a prolonged period of time.[17] It's not for nothing that in yoga, erect standing positions such as the "warrior poses" are used for the purpose of increasing power and alertness. The fact that posture has an effect on the psyche also becomes apparent in laughter yoga. Even when people laugh without any humor and only grimace, their mood is improved. It follows that stretching your back after waking up and smiling at yourself in the mirror can have the same effect as medicine.

As a doctor who has worked in intensive care units and ambulances, I saw the effects of prolonged daily stress: Stress was almost always involved when younger people suffered from heart problems, hypertensive crises, or asthma attacks. During my night shifts, heart attack patients told me stories of family and marital problems or financial worries, all of which severely depressed them. It's very rare for stress alone to cause an acute heart attack. But stress can cause heart attacks in the long run, and it also intensifies many additional adverse factors. If you're under stress, you likely also exercise less, eat too quickly and less healthy, smoke and drink more, and suffer from sleep disorders.

Time and again it's been confirmed in many conversations with patients that stress contributes to hypertension, asthma, irritable bowel syndrome and inflammations of the bowel, many skin disorders, head and back pain, as well as rheumatism and other autoimmune diseases and allergies, because stressed nerves communicate with the immune cells and disturb the signaling molecules and messenger cycles, i.e., our internal survival chemistry. A large-scale study from 2017 also proved that stress heightens the risk of cancer. Cancer of the pancreas, the large intestine, the esophagus, and the prostate occurs two to four times more often in people who have stated earlier that they were under a great amount of stress.[18]

Scientific research on stress began in the beginning of the twentieth century. Walter Cannon, physiologist at Harvard University, explained the body's responses to stress as a "fight or flight reaction," an immensely important survival strategy. When under threat, muscles tense, heartbeat and blood pressure increase, perception turns to tunnel vision, and the body tries to get rid of unnecessary weight—the contents of bladder and bowel—one is literally "scared shitless."

This reflex enabled our primeval ancestors to either take flight or stand and fight. That way, one could escape the danger—or face it head on. But stress in the workplace or worries about the future don't cease to exist after a sprint or a short battle. They have the tendency to become chronic, and therefore there is also no period of relaxation. Instead, we suffer from back pains, hypertension, heart attacks, and depressions.

Occasional "doses" of stress can potentially strengthen body and mind—you can experience personal growth after a difficult calamity because that's when we develop resilience, the ability to withstand the blows of fate. This is a training effect similar to that achieved by exercise, Scotch hose treatments, or fasting, but on a psychological level. When you ask people about their life crises, interestingly it becomes obvious that it's not those who have had no negative experiences at all who are doing the best, but those who have lived through a certain number of crises and trauma. That said, everyone has a tipping point, at which the initially increasing performance ability begins to decrease because the exertion is too great.

Stress hormones cause blood vessels to constrict, blood pressure to rise, and the hands to become cold, as well as the tip of the nose in

## How Stress Affects the Body

- Fosters depression, anxiety, and sleep disorders
- Accelerates breathing
- Heightens levels of blood sugar, insulin, and blood fats
- Fosters blood clots
- Heightens muscle tension and reduces bone density
- Impairs memory and concentration
- Narrows thoughts, causes headaches
- Increases heart rate and blood pressure
- Diminishes nutrient uptake and disrupts digestion
- Impairs immune function
- Aggravates obesity
- Leads to infertility

some instances. My former boss in the cardiology department used to touch the tip of the nose of severely ill patients in the ICU: If it was cold, it meant that the situation was rather critical.

At the naturopathic hospital in Essen, I used biodots for the first time; they are pea-sized dots that are stuck to the back of the hand. Via thermal sensors, they indicate body temperature and illustrate in which situations stress occurs. I remember one patient, a top executive with hypertension and a sleep disorder. I had expected that he would be tense due to his undoubtedly exhausting line of work—but the biodots revealed something else entirely: At work, his hands were being supplied with blood sufficiently, but at home his vessels constricted, possibly because he was suffering from a guilty conscience since he could only spend such little time with his family. The executive hadn't expected this, either. A lot of the time, stress is misjudged the same way relaxation is misjudged: Many people believe, for instance, that they are relaxing when they watch television, but usually the opposite is the case.

We see then that a temporary strain activates the immune system. But this effect is quickly depleted if the stress persists. That's why we are easy prey for viral infections when we are sleep-deprived and

exhausted. Wound repair is also impaired and takes longer. This realization is slowly asserting itself among surgeons—some patients get to
listen to CDs with relaxing music before an operation. Should you
have to undergo surgery, you should perform a deep relaxation session
every day of the week before the appointment.[19] Meditation is best or,
alternatively, there is autogenic training. Yoga exercises are ideal to
stretch the fasciae and keep them supple. In addition, it would be helpful to fast for a couple of days beforehand (as long as you are not un-
derweight). By the way, music in the OR, regardless of whether you are
under general anesthesia or not, reduces fear. As a consequence, less
pain medication is necessary.[20, 21]

To summarize the results of the numerous studies, the following
risk factors for sickening stress emerge:

- a heavy workload in conjunction with little decision-making
  power
- marriage or relationship problems
- arguments with family or friends
- caring for a relative
- experiences of violence and abuse as a child
- symptoms of a disease (particularly pain)
- sleep deprivation and not enough periods of rest
- the feeling that the strain being experienced is meaningless

## MIND-BODY MEDICINE: BRINGING BODY, MIND, AND SOUL IN HARMONY

What do we do with these findings? It's hardly possible to lead a life
without stress—this is the starting point from where many Eastern
philosophies begin. As the Buddha said: Life is pain. Surely, one

ought to reduce objective stress factors and make life easy, but usually that is not possible without fundamentally changing one's coordinate system.

This is where mind-body medicine comes in—a further development of naturopathic organizational therapy. While it deals with the traditional pillars of a healthy lifestyle—more physical activity, a better diet, and sufficient relaxation—mind-body medicine is predominantly focused on having a positive effect on the interrelationships between the psyche, the immune system, and the nervous system. To achieve that, it exercises mental techniques and implements behavioral changes. In that way it supports our body's abilities of self-regulation and self-healing.

In therapeutic practice, mind-body medicine draws on elements of traditional healing methods like yoga, tai chi, qigong, or meditation, but also on modern relaxation methods and mindfulness techniques, such as progressive muscle relaxation. At the naturopathic hospital in Essen as well as at the Immanuel Hospital in Berlin, mind-body teams work with patients on developing individual strategies they can implement after their discharge from the clinic—in order to transfer the successes achieved during their treatment to their daily lives. The therapists are nutritionists, meditation and yoga instructors, sports scientists, social workers, or psychologists. To me, mind-body medicine is the key to a sustainable effect. Because not only does it counteract stress as an important risk factor, it also helps patients perceive their body in a new way and start taking responsibility for it.

All traditional healing systems ascribe great importance to the connection between mind and body. With the scientific foundation of medicine in the modern age, however, many of these connections have taken a back seat. Suddenly, mind and body were considered separate entities. Only stress research, psychosomatics, and psychoneuroimmunology engaged with the complex relationships between body, soul, and the nervous system. Like the American rheumatologist George Solomon, who in the 1960s discovered that rheumatoid arthritis worsened when the patients were suffering from depression at the same time. He began to examine the correlation between inflammatory diseases, the immune system, and emotions.[22]

To accommodate ideas like this, the cardiologist Herbert Benson developed a new way of looking at cardiovascular diseases in the 1970s: He did not focus on the organ, but on the emotions that make it sick. It should be possible, Benson thought, to reverse the body's reactions to stress—to turn the chain reaction of the fight-or-flight impulse into relaxation. He noted the positive effect meditation had on the nervous system and from that he derived a series of relaxation techniques that slow down the heartbeat, lower the blood pressure, and relax the muscles.[23] He founded the Benson-Henry Institute for Mind Body Medicine at the Harvard Medical School and has remained one of the most important pioneers in mind-body medicine to this day.

By now, all major hospitals and universities in the United States have their own departments of mind-body medicine. The National Center for Complementary and Integrative Health (NCCIH), part of the national health authority, considers mind-body medicine as an independent component of complementary medicine and supports research projects in this field.

Quite often, experiences from the past—as far back as childhood—come up in conversations with patients. These experiences, if dealt with consciously, constitute an important step toward convalescence. Mind-body medicine, however, goes a step further—or rather, backward. Instead of talking about their past experiences, patients are placed in a room in which they can heal themselves in a "prelinguistic" way, through relaxation, silence, and mindfulness. This sounds esoteric, but it's not: A lot of recent scientific data proves in an impressive way how effective mind-body techniques are, especially in the treatment of chronic diseases.

Each of these techniques has specific characteristics—not all of them work in the same way and are equally suitable for everyone. For some, qigong, the Chinese moving meditation, is too boring. Others find yoga too athletic or they can't manage staying in the meditation posture for long. Therefore, you cannot "prescribe" mind-body medicine, you can only demonstrate it and encourage practice. The patients should find techniques that they can easily integrate into their daily routine because there is one unpleasant feature of mind-body medicine: For it to work, it has to be practiced regularly. In the following sections, you'll find suggestions to inspire you.

## YOGA: INDIA'S GIFT TO THE WORLD

Yoga is booming. These days you can find a yoga studio in every major American city. The 2016 Yoga in America study commissioned by the *Yoga Journal* and Yoga Alliance estimated that more than 36 million people practice yoga in the United States.

Yoga is more than two thousand years old. The word *yoga* itself comes from Sanskrit, the original language of the literature and philosophy of India. It goes back to the root *yui* and means to meet, to unite, or to gather the mind. One way of interpreting this is as the body and the consciousness becoming one. Traditional yoga is actually not concerned with therapeutic effects, but rather with reaching a mental and spiritual (nonreligious) goal. The medical effects, however, are an important and useful side effect.

Indians proudly say that yoga was India's gift to the world. On the initiative of the Indian government and Prime Minister Narendra

Modi, himself a practitioner of yoga, the United Nations declared June 21 to be International Day of Yoga in 2015. Modi has even appointed a minister of yoga, who is also responsible for Ayurveda and other traditional healing methods.

Yoga has been examined by science for more than fifteen years and has turned out to be an exceedingly successful therapy—in an unambiguity that has surprised even myself. That said, only a small portion of it is practiced and researched in the West. In my generation, many people set out for India after their university studies or their apprenticeship and went on the legendary hippie trail. Often, the goal was Northern India, holy cities like Rishikesh or Haridwar, where one center for meditation and yoga (ashram) followed the other. And so, it didn't take long for yoga to reach Europe and America. Maybe you'll be able to find the book *Yoga for Everyone* by the Canadian yoga teacher Kareen Zebroff at a flea market. Today it's become a classic; back then, in the '70s, it was the first attempt at translating yoga poses into an easily practicable training program.

In the year 2000 I was ready, too. It was a morning, while I was at the new department for naturopathy at the hospitals in Essen-Mitte. I had slept badly, work just wouldn't end, and my back was aching. I knew that when I slept restlessly and had a lot of stress, my back acted up. Otto Langels, the new director of nursing and a passionate disciple of yoga, took one critical look at me and said: "You really ought to go to a yoga class!" At first, I didn't take him seriously—when you're not doing too well, you don't want to be lectured. But since the pain wouldn't let up, I sheepishly visited the yoga class as he had suggested—one that followed the teachings of the yoga guru B. K. S. Iyengar.

To my great surprise, those ninety minutes of my life had noticeable consequences: I left with really sore muscles—muscles that I had never felt before and of whose existence I only knew from my anatomy classes at university—and my back pain was gone. I hadn't expected it to work so immediately. In the following years I've been able to observe this time and again. As soon as I stop going to yoga, my back pain returns. I do yoga exercises—and hey, presto!—the pain is gone.

## YOGA GIVES YOU ENERGY, REDUCES STRESS, AND RELIEVES PAIN

Almost all participants of the yoga classes I went to had the same experience I did: After a session you feel more energetic, and your mood improves. Yoga gives you energy immediately and does so at an astonishing speed, which I had never found in other forms of exercise in the same fashion. And so, in 2003, I began planning a scientific study on yoga and its effects on stress. We placed an ad looking for participants who were feeling stressed. To my great surprise more than 90 percent of the people who got in touch were women. Many of them were single parents and had an exhausting daily routine.

We decided to conduct the experiment exclusively with women under heavy strain and divided them into two groups. One group received the offer of visiting a ninety-minute Iyengar yoga class one or two times a week for free over the course of three months. We asked the other group to wait, and promised them the same offer once the three months were up. During this period we ascertained their stress level, mental state, and the cortisol levels in their saliva (the cortisol level was actually measured after every single yoga class).

The results were impressive. Yoga led to a pronounced lowering of stress level. Overall mood was improved, as were anxiety and depressiveness. But not only that—many of the participants stated that their head and back pains were reduced to a dramatic extent. For most, even a single class caused a significant lowering of stress hormones. We published this (still small) study and continued with another, bigger study with seventy-two participants.[24, 25]

This time we were interested in whether practicing more yoga could potentially have an even greater effect. We randomly divided women into three groups. One group was asked to do ninety minutes of yoga once a week, the second twice as much, and the third was once again asked to wait. The result was that the first two groups showed similar effects. It's likely that more yoga didn't lead to more effectiveness because for many of the women it simply wasn't possible to take two classes a week, and they felt additional stress because of our request.

We can conclude that yoga is an excellent remedy for stress and that ninety minutes a week is sufficient. And of course, it's not a bad thing to take out the yoga mat at home every once in a while. But do go to a class. Patients often ask me if they couldn't teach themselves—with YouTube, a DVD, or a book. No. The danger of getting into the habit of doing an exercise, a pose, the wrong way is too big, and this can lead to incorrect weight placement or even injury.

Over the following years, research findings kept appearing in quick succession. Particularly where my personal weak spot, back pain, was concerned, numerous studies have proved how efficient yoga is—more effective than most other therapies, that is.[26] In cooperation with the Berlin-based Iyengar Institute, we were able to show the same result for chronic neck pain in 2012.[27] Other studies have demonstrated the effectiveness of yoga for headaches, hypertension, and soft tissue rheumatism. Yoga also led to the notable relief of symptoms of chronic inflammatory bowel disease according to the findings of our colleagues in Essen.[28]

## YOGA SUPPORTS CANCER TREATMENT

What is most impressive to me is that yoga is also effective as a supplementary therapy for cancer. American researchers were able to prove that women suffering from breast cancer experienced a remarkable increase in their quality of life when they went to yoga classes for serval weeks.[29] Up until now, there has been no better remedy against the frequent fatigue and severe tiredness that can occur during and after a cancer treatment and that heavily restricts the patient's daily life.

A research team in Essen headed by psychologist Holger Cramer has published many meta-studies on the effectiveness of yoga.[30, 31, 32] The list of successes spans from menopausal symptoms to complimentary treatment of heart diseases and hypertension. Even atrial fibrillation, a cardiac arrhythmia that is difficult to control with medication, is alleviated. There is hardly any area of medicine in which yoga isn't useful.

Among the abundance of yoga classes out there, it can be difficult to find the right one. Unfortunately, the term "yoga instructor" isn't protected. It can mean anything from an intensive training program over the course of many years or just a three-week course. The Iyengar school, however, is quite thorough. I can recommend it. It also works with props like blocks and straps. Iyengar-yoga instructors have definitely undergone several years of training, and for medicinal yoga therapy there are even higher requirements that must be met.

## WHAT KIND OF YOGA IS SUITABLE FOR YOU

Where other schools are concerned, it's important to make sure that they are recognized by the Yoga Alliance. This is a certain seal of quality. Still, the standards should be defined better. There are many good yoga schools, from Iyengar to Ashtanga, from Kundalini to Vini, from Sivananda to Vinyasa—but not everything suits everyone. Use trial lessons to figure out which kind of yoga agrees with you!

Some people fear that there are religious or esoteric elements in yoga. I can reassure you there. The prayer position of the hands and the chanting of Om aren't necessarily to be equated with religious practice but are merely a part of Hindu tradition. In India, a guru isn't the leader of a sect, but a teacher (one who is certainly highly revered). If you want to avoid spiritual connotations, you should learn Iyengar yoga, since it's quite sober and focused on the body. The rooms usually look like they would in a practice for physical therapy. For yoga, you need neither incense nor a Buddha statue, just two square meters to roll out a yoga mat. That's what makes it so appealing to me. Once you know how it's done, you can practice it at home easily. It's cheap and effective.

People with medical problems should choose their yoga practice especially carefully. For example, Bikram Hot Yoga, which involves great exertion in rooms at temperatures of 104 degrees, isn't suitable for people with health problems. Patients with rheumatism or arthritis, particularly those with damaged knees or menisci, have to tread particularly carefully and should consult an experienced yoga instructor. In 2012, the American journalist William J. Broad published the *New York Times* best seller *The Science of Yoga: Risks and Rewards*. In it, the danger of injury from doing yoga was discussed for the first time. People with hypermobility, a genetically determined excessive flexibility of the joints, for instance, should refrain from doing yoga or only practice it under the supervision of very experienced instructors. Similarly, some yoga poses are unsuitable for people suffering from glaucoma, i.e., increased pressure in the eye. But the general rule is that yoga is just as safe and carries as few side effects as normal physical therapy and mild exercise. Remember to pay attention to your body's signals when doing yoga. It's not about doing the headstand come what may or reaching your hands as low as you can toward the ground. First and foremost, it's about being aware of your body.

If it were up to me, I would integrate yoga into school sports. It's a method of movement that can be practiced for a lifetime without any great effort and that doesn't cause what school sports normally lead to— frustration. You don't have to achieve great performances. We are just now testing this in a study with students at a trade school. Yoga is well received, reduces stress, and promotes well-being even in adolescents.

## WHAT MAKES YOGA SO SPECIAL

How can yoga be superior to exercise in some areas? Possibly, yoga is so special because it combines five different elements:

- It strengthens the muscles.
- It connects body coordination to breathing—competitive athletes know how important this is in order to achieve the optimal effect through the interaction of body and circulation.
- It leads to deep relaxation—most of all during Shavasana (corpse pose), usually the position that marks the end of a session.
- It stretches the body thoroughly, leading to the release of endorphins and thereby calming the autonomic nervous system, which is of immense importance. In a study, U.S. scientists conducted an initial comparison between yoga and physical therapy to treat back pain and discovered that yoga was superior to physical therapy. In a second study, they added intensive, yoga-like

stretching exercises to the physical therapy. After that, it was almost as good as yoga.[33, 34]

- Yoga has an effect on the fasciae. With its particular mixture of extending, stretching, and reversing, yoga relaxes and maintains the connective tissue and the fasciae.

## THE EIGHT STEPS TO YOGA

In the West, we usually have the physical poses (*asanas*) in mind when we think of yoga. According to traditional teachings, however, there are eight steps that make up yoga in its entirety. For instance, breathing exercises (*pranayama*) can have in-depth effects on the body via the autonomic nervous system—such as cooling down the body in great heat or warming it up when it's cold. There are special exercises for almost every objective. By now it has been proven that pranayama techniques have a profound effect on lung volume in chronic obstructive pulmonary disease (COPD), that they stabilize the heart rhythm and can even influence gene expression rather swiftly.[35] The latter means that inflammations are reduced on a molecular level. Proteins that contribute to diseases such as diabetes and arteriosclerosis are produced less, even though such epigenetic phenomena can usually only be induced with medication. It must be noted, however, that most studies examine the combination of asanas and pranayama, so that it's not possible to accurately determine which of the two has the healing effect.

I have experienced firsthand how strong an effect breathing can have. A yoga instructor showed me activating breathing exercises, among them the so-called bellows-breathing (*bhastrika pranayama*). I was excited. The next evening, I was feeling a little exhausted after work and started doing this and other exercises at great speed over the course of forty-five minutes. In the beginning, I felt in top shape and highly alert. But the "reckoning" followed soon: At night I slept quite restlessly, and by the afternoon of the next day I was lying in bed with a cold. Instead of listening to my exhaustion and relaxing, I had started a fire inside my body.

Furthermore, the withdrawal of the senses (*pratyahara*) and concentration (*dharana*) belong to the eight-step path of yoga. The Indian scholar Patanjali, who authored the guidelines of yoga, so to say, sometime between the second century BCE and the fourth century CE, perceived focusing as the most important element: "Yoga is the ability to focus the mind exclusively towards an object and sustain that direction without any distraction."

Another step is self-discipline (*niyama*), which includes bodily hygiene as well as the development of a culture of contentedness and a healthy lifestyle. The moral basis is *yamas*, consideration for other living beings, which also includes the recommendation for a vegetarian lifestyle. The aim of physical exercises mainly consists of being able to devote oneself to sitting in meditation (*dhyana*) for as long as possible which then (potentially) leads to smadhi, the unity of everything and a superconscious experience. It needs to be emphasized that yoga is not a religion.

## YOGA: OFTEN MORE EFFECTIVE THAN EXERCISE AND PHYSICAL THERAPY

I practice yoga regularly and yet I still find myself amazed at how the different poses can lead to different physical effects. Bending forward tends to be calming, while bending backward is strongly stimulating and makes you alert. There are exercises that facilitate sleep and some that prevent it. This is something we don't find in our Western sports, and modern science is unable to explain this with hormones and molecules alone. Another unique feature of yoga is the enormous delicacy and precision of body postures and movements. The technical term is "alignment." Every millimeter is counted for, and the fine tuning is of a precision that our European physical therapy lacks.

Yoga is therefore also applied anatomy. So, it's all the more surprising that this knowledge of muscles, tendons, ligaments, fasciae, and organs already existed before anatomical knowledge was garnered from corpses at a much later stage. On a visit to India I once witnessed this astonishing skill: B. K. S. Iyengar showed me a patient who was having trouble breathing after bypass surgery. My first thought as a doctor was that the bypasses had closed again. But that wasn't the case. Iyengar palpated the patient and determined that his ribs were blocked after the intense surgical intervention, and the scar allowed only for very shallow breathing movements in the chest. With targeted instructions, he showed the patient how to stretch the ribs wider in order to use the whole chest for breathing. The respiratory problems were resolved quickly.

By the way, a study conducted by the Technical University of Munich from 2000 to 2005 with approximately one thousand heart attack patients showed that patients who were breathing faster after a heart attack had a bigger risk of dying earlier.[36] Yoga or meditation can lower quickness of breath.

Iyengar yoga has an excellent effect in women who have undergone treatment for breast cancer. It's possible that this may be the result of something similar to the Iyengar example with the bypass patient. Surgery, radiation, and chemotherapy compromise physical feeling and thus the flexibility of the ribs. With yoga, the chest and breathing can be freed, and a pleasant physical feeling can be restored.

An article in *GEO* magazine on the Iyengar school was entitled "Pain Is Your Master." The article was published in 1990 and has often been misinterpreted. The intention is not for yoga to cause pain, but to

teach us to feel the limits of endurance. When stretching or reinforcing muscles we may experience some pain. But this pain, which in
naturopathy we call "the good pain," is different from the kind of pain
that causes us suffering. Some massage and physical therapy techniques work with dosed and controlled pain, as do acupuncture and
cupping to a certain degree. Yoga helps us find sensation and mindfulness, it uses the "body's intelligence," as Iyengar described it.

When I look at the scientific data on yoga—at its great effectiveness and safety—it remains incomprehensible why there aren't more
hospitals that offer yoga, and more health insurance companies that
bear the costs for it. In Germany, it's possible to be partially reimbursed for one's expenses for yoga classes from health insurance companies as part of a prevention measure. But the use of yoga lies
pre-eminently in therapy, not just in prevention. In any case, there is
no rational reason to reimburse the costs of orthopedic injections and
all kinds of surgeries while the equally effective, if not superior, yoga
has to be paid for out of one's own pocket.

## MEDITATION: THE ART OF INNER REFLECTION, OF CALM, OF NOT THINKING

I had my first practical experience with meditation during my mind-
body training with Herbert Benson at Harvard Medical School. My
initiation, however, wasn't exactly laudable. Peg Baim, Benson's meditation expert, asked us to pay attention to our breath and not to let
thoughts disturb the silence. When thoughts arose, we were to wel-
come them—and then send them off again. In no way were we to lin-
ger on them. Rather, we were meant to simply send these thoughts on
their way.

This was difficult for me, since I was and continue to be in a line of work that requires a lot of thinking. I was sitting on my chair (it's not mandatory to sit on the floor) and tried to focus on my breath. After three or four minutes my thoughts had calmed down somewhat, but suddenly a strong feeling of fear arose within me. I was about to quit and leave the room, but that was too embarrassing for me, so I tried to conquer my fear. After a while the panic disappeared, and it has never returned during any of my sessions of meditating.

It's not unusual for fear to arise during the first attempts at meditation. Having to deal with emptiness all of a sudden is probably strange for the brain. The consciously chosen experience of quiet is a key component of meditation. It is an interruption of our permanently flowing stream of thoughts. Some irreverently call this automatized activity of the brain the "madhouse" or the "autopilot." For most people it's a completely unexpected realization to see how hard it is *not* to think.

In its Latin origin, *meditatio* means "to center toward the middle." It's a return to a prelinguistic experience. All of us were conscious before we learned to speak. But as soon as language arrived, it dominated everything. And as successful as it is in shaping our lives, it can interfere with relaxation and calmness. As early as two decades ago, stress researchers pointed out that it's not only situations that are exhausting—thinking about them is just as exhausting.[37] And so, it's possible for the memory of a trauma to elicit a physical response. Worries, brooding, and a merry-go-round of thoughts can place the body in a state of constant stress. And our endless stream of thoughts don't necessarily even lead to a solution, as many problems can't be solved by thinking alone. Herein also lies the central difference to psychotherapy or to conversations: Meditation begins before language. Through silence and not thinking we can reach realizations that wouldn't be possible to reach by thinking. In the quiet, our brain seems to be able to find solutions via paths that would normally be closed off by the constant stream of thoughts.

All forms of meditation incorporate the knowledge that it's extremely hard for people not to think. To make it easier, various aids are used, such as monotonous word sequences—mantras—that are employed mainly to busy our restless mind. You repeat them and concentrate on, for example, the colors or images that appear in front of your closed eyes at the same time. Zen meditation attempts to gather the concentration, for example, by focusing on looking at a candle. Another Zen technique consists of paradoxical thought experiments, the *kōans*, which are puzzles that cannot be solved by rational thinking; only through prolonged meditation can a different understanding be reached.

Scientific research into mind-body medicine, by the way, has used transcendental meditation as a starting point, which is why its effects on the body have been well-examined (the lowering of blood pressure, the reduction of stress, and the relief from pain). Still, I don't recommend it, because a lot of money is asked for the transfer of a mantra. This contradicts meditation as it is practiced in Indian yoga.

## MINDFULNESS: THE RECIPE FOR STRESS REDUCTION

Over the past ten years, mindfulness meditation has spread widely. Here, you're not concentrating on anything nor are you repeating any specific words; you are silent and aware. You are aware of what is happening in the body, in your thoughts and feelings—without judging anything. Mindfulness meditation was developed further and introduced to medicine by the molecular biologist and stress researcher Jon Kabat-Zinn. To free it from its religious references and thus make it accessible to everybody, he stripped it of its Buddhist and spiritual approaches. That way, this secularized form of meditation was able to spread around the globe.

It uses mainly two techniques: In one technique, the entire body is palpated from head to toe, like in a CT scan, in what is called a body scan, but not in a mechanical and imaging way, but with the aid of perception. Therefore, it is possible for you to feel where a pain is actually located and what it feels like exactly for the first time. But it's also possible that pleasant physical feelings are perceived through this exercise for the first time. In the other technique of mindfulness meditation, awareness is directed toward the breath. Any thoughts that pop into your head are named, such as financial worries or disputes in the family, in order to then separate yourself from your thoughts.

Based on this, Kabat-Zinn developed an eight-week training program, the Mindfulness-Based Stress Reduction Program (MBSR). Over the course of these eight weeks, the participants are asked to perform certain meditative exercises for forty-five minutes every day. This commitment is worth it: A considerable number of studies have been able to prove the great effectiveness of MBSR in the treatment of many chronic diseases. They show a clear healing effect or at least a relief of the symptoms in chronic back pain, depression, and stress.[38] In mild and moderate depressions, mindfulness meditation is just as effective as antidepressants.[39] And in very severe, incurable diseases like cancer or multiple sclerosis, it's truly beneficial. The interruption of thoughts enables patients to push aside their anxieties about the future and return to the present, to the moment. That's when they often find that their condition is not actually that bad. This in turn can reduce tension, relieve pain, and improve the functioning of the immune system.[40]

In fact, one of the most exciting effects of meditation is that though pain doesn't actually disappear, it is perceived as less debilitating. To demonstrate this, researchers inflicted a pain stimulus—the prick of a needle or heat—on test subjects and subsequently examined the activation of pain centers in the brain in an MRI scanner. People who had been meditating regularly showed only half of the amount of pain center activation in the brain. It follows that meditation not only enables people to deal with pain better, but even leads to a real reduction of pain perception in the brain—the actual place from which pain originates.[41]

Meditation is very soothing, particularly with incurable, chronic diseases since it trains us to accept symptoms that cannot be eliminated through therapy. And the fact that lifelong complete health is not attainable for most people is what makes meditation so valuable. It's not for nothing that Kabat-Zinn entitled his first book *Full Catastrophe Living*. Chaos, sorrow, and illness are a part of life. Meditation can help us learn to be happy in spite of this realization.

## DISTANCING YOURSELF FROM YOUR SUFFERING

I first met Jon Kabat-Zinn in 1999. Gustav Dobos had invited him to the naturopathic hospital in Essen to lead a training course. We rented a school gym and meditated in a group for several sessions, each thirty to forty-five minutes. The course was interspersed with presentations and discussions of scientific findings on psoriasis, fibromyalgia, or post-traumatic stress disorder. It was a cheerful, inspiring atmosphere and our guest didn't even let on that he was jetlagged. When the event came to its close, we were determined to introduce mindfulness meditation as a therapeutic method at our hospital in Essen.

The most important action to undertake in meditation is distancing oneself from one's own suffering. The technical term for this is metacognition—taking the position of an observer, like seeing the world from a bird's-eye perspective. From my own experiences with meditation I know this: If you truly commit to it, you can free yourself from even the gravest worries and distance yourself from what is bothering you. Of course, pain and grief remain, but they don't drain you of your energy so much.

Another big advantage that comes from meditation is becoming less judgmental. Usually, we immediately attach a feeling, often a negative one, to everything that happens. When you see the brake lights of the car in front of you on the highway light up, you automatically start "catastrophizing": Is there an accident ahead? How long am I going to be stuck in traffic? What happens if I don't get to my destination on time? And so on. When you meditate regularly, non-judging is reinforced. Non-judging helps in our communication with others, because you no longer try and comment on everything straight away, but rather just perceive things as they are for the time being. Even when you feel anger, you don't lose control but seek to observe, occupying a position of insight.

And finally, mindfulness is connected to basic virtues: a curious attitude, compassion, empathy, joy, and patience.

For people who put emphasis on their body, focusing on the breath is the best way to get started. For people who have a hard time relaxing, it can be helpful to name occurring thoughts before dismissing them, or visualize putting those thoughts in a drawer. Those interested in spirituality might want to try Vipassana meditation.

I chose to follow a mystic meditation from India, a mantra meditation where you close your eyes and concentrate on what you see and on the images that appear. We conducted two studies on this Iyoti meditation. A few patients with neck pain that had persisted for ten years on average were instructed in this type of meditation, others were asked to wait. After two months it became apparent that the group that meditated was experiencing significantly less pain, even though their limited mobility had not disappeared—this, in turn, showed that meditation is a way of influencing the brain, not a method of miraculous healing.

A multitude of studies on meditation have produced fascinating results. The team around Herbert Benson, for example, was able to document in 2013 that regular mindfulness meditation has a favorable influence on gene expression even after a relatively short period of practicing it.[42] Other researchers proved that telomerase activity can be improved through meditation—telomerase are the enzymes that repair genetic material.[43] Additionally, brain research was able to demonstrate that meditation is linked to an increase in the density of gray matter in the areas responsible for learning, emotions, and perspective thinking.[44]

Studies have shown that meditation is superior to most other relaxation methods, such as progressive muscle relaxation.[45] Though patients often prefer progressive muscle relaxation because it only takes a short time, where hypertension is concerned it is defeated by the positive effects of meditation. Meditation is simply the most effective method of mind-body medicine.

Take your time—it's worth sticking with it. In mindfulness-based stress reduction (MBSR) you should meditate for forty-five minutes every day (including doing the body scan). In transcendental meditation it's forty minutes, and in Iyoti meditation it's thirty to sixty minutes. For those who can't sit still for that long I recommend going jogging or doing yoga beforehand and then meditating afterward, into the period of relaxation.

There are four reasons why it's worthwhile to meditate:

1. Meditation causes the "relaxation response" in the body and does so in the most effective way compared to other methods.

2. The brain responds to meditation to such an extent that you almost get the impression that the body has been waiting for this specific program. Meditation and yoga help us find balance in our severely accelerated lives. The enormous concentration on spoken activity has largely replaced physical work, thoughts "tower" in our heads, and stress hormones can no longer be reduced. Meditation offers a way of creating a balance here.

3. Meditation sharpens our ability to concentrate and focus. Some may find the fact that companies use meditation to increase efficiency to be in bad taste. There's nothing wrong with that, but it's not its original purpose.

4. And finally, there is the path to spirituality, which is connected to questions about our existence and the purpose of life. It is a yearning for answers that most people experience, no matter whether they are religious or not. Even atheists can devote themselves to these issues in meditation. Meditation is medication for the soul, wrote the renowned meditation teacher Rajinder Singh.[46] Perceiving the limitations of our individual agency can have a comforting effect in the way we approach our everyday lives. "Everybody has to die, maybe even I," the German comedian Karl Valentin, a hypochondriac, once said.

So try to learn meditation, either in person or following a video or audio recording. Try to find time for it on a regular basis—this, sadly, is where I fail from time to time, but that's life. Mornings are better than evenings, because the brain is not quite so overloaded yet. You'll be better prepared for a busy day and will suffer less stress. Meditate for thirty minutes, maybe half as long in the beginning, but then you should seek to continuously increase the duration. Find a seated position in which you feel as comfortable as possible—in no way does it have to be the lotus position. You can also sit straight on a chair. Get ready, get set, go: Don't wait—meditate.

## BREATHING SLOWLY PROLONGS YOUR LIFE

Both *pranayama* (yogic breathing) and meditation cause us to breathe a little slower (which, coincidentally, is also a positive result of endurance sports). Normally, we breathe fifteen times a minute. Under stress and physical exertion that number is higher. Many yoga and qigong exercises aim to reduce this frequency to six breaths a minute. This leads to a slower pulse and is supposedly very healthy for the heart, the blood vessels, and the organs. Ancient yoga texts claim that everyone has a predetermined number of breaths. You may dismiss this as a mystic legend, but what's interesting is that slow breathing, particularly in patients with heart disease, is actually connected to a longer lifespan.

In general, meditation leads to slower breathing. A similar effect is achieved by prayer. That's why, according to the American concept of mind-body medicine, prayer is a part of meditation. This may cause some furrowed brows—prayer as part of medical therapy? People pray for a variety of reasons, usually not to treat hypertension or headaches. But nevertheless it has a positive effect on our health. Of course, people with no religious background are unlikely to start praying solely for therapeutic reasons. But if you are already doing it, you can be happy about the fact that it also has a medicinal effect.

One of the researchers who published particularly impressive findings on the matter is the Italian physiologist and internist Luciano Bernardi at the University of Padua. He and his team have conducted research into the positive effects of slow breathing. In a couple of studies, they were able to prove that breathing according to ancient yoga techniques—wherein only six breaths are taken a minute—leads to positive effects in patients suffering from cardiac insufficiency. These people often breathe very fast in their desire to get more air, but this causes their breaths to be shallow. Many times, the shallow flow of air is not enough to achieve the necessary interchange of gases in the pulmonary alveoli, i.e., the coupling of oxygen to the red blood cells. As a consequence, they breathe even faster because they feel a shortness of breath.

Bernardi and his colleagues demonstrated that oxygen content in the blood increases as soon as patients are instructed to breathe calmly and slowly. Inspired by this observation they began to take an interest in other techniques of prayer and meditation, including those that work with mantras, the slow and repeated sequences of words. Many meditation techniques that employ mantras have been developed in Asia; in the Catholic Christian tradition there is the rosary prayer, which consists of periodic repetitions of word sequences, so-called decades. In the rosary, each prayer cycle is said over the course of one breath that lasts for about ten seconds—this comes out to six breaths a minute, which aligns with the six breaths of yoga. Bernardi and his team studied the rhythms of the pulse rate and the breath as well as the delicate coordination by the autonomic nervous system in three situations: having participants recite the Ave Maria in Latin, having participants recite the ancient Tibetan mantra "*om mani padme hum,*" and having participants speak normally.

Interestingly, reciting both the Ave Maria and the Tibetan mantra led to a breathing sequence of six breaths a minute as well as an astonishing synchronization and thus an improvement of heart, lung, and breathing rhythms. Even blood pressure and heart rate were lowered, and the cerebral blood flow improved. When speaking normally, however, the study participants took in more than twice as many breaths—fourteen times a minute.[47]

The repetition of religious prayers and mantras seem to have profoundly beneficial effects on our body. But it's not just praying that is healthy—regular visits to church have a positive effect on our health, too, according to the findings of the largest study as of yet on the matter, published in 2016 in *JAMA Internal Medicine*. In the Nurses' Health Study, the health and disease development of roughly 75,000 nurses was documented continuously over a period of sixteen years. During that time there were 13,500 deaths. After risk factors like smoking, high cholesterol levels, or insufficient exercise were excluded statistically, it became apparent that women who visited mass at least once a week had a death rate that was 33 percent lower than the average. This was especially significant in heart diseases, where the death rate was 38 percent lower, but also in cancer diseases (27 percent less). The researchers were unable to explain what exactly had caused this phenomenon. But it wasn't just the solidarity within the congregation, the social factor. Maybe it was a trust in God that manifested itself in greater serenity.[48]

Unsurprisingly, people—religious or not—usually begin to pray when they are going through hardship, when they have grave sorrows. Intuitively, this relieves the stress they are under in that situation. Trust in God and church attendance probably also help against depression. Areas of the brain that are connected to positive moods show greater resonance in these instances. Though doctors certainly won't prescribe a visit to church, for people who are already religious or practice spirituality it can constitute a further health-promoting reinforcement.

# CHAPTER EIGHT

# Global Medicines

*Ayurveda, Acupuncture, and the Healing Power of Plants*

t was the year 2006 and I found myself, still in Essen at the time, in a period of upheaval. I had just finished a study on yoga with impressive results, and from the growing success that mind-body medicine had in my patients it was foreseeable that meditation, which I was practicing with increasing enthusiasm, was the supreme discipline among the different relaxation methods and mental techniques. This shifted my focus increasingly eastward.

Up until that point, I had never been to India, and maybe that is why I realized quite late, but all the more intensely, that this country was an important birthplace of naturopathic medicine. After all, I had already developed a strong interest in Ayurveda—particularly within the scope of comparative traditional medicine that spanned the cultural areas of Europe, China, Tibet, and India. In doing so, some remarkable analogies had become apparent. Ayurveda, I noted, is among those healing methods that focus on the individual and is based on constitutional types. Beyond that, traditional Indian medicine emphasizes prevention, lifestyle, and self-efficacy. It has developed techniques that aren't merely targeted at symptoms, but at an internal power balance. If necessary, eliminating methods like bloodletting and leeches are employed. Ayurveda possesses a range of healing methods and aims for the activation of self-healing powers. Just as in European naturopathy, chronic diseases and functional disruptions are the focus. What's particularly great about Ayurveda is that it's an undogmatic healing system and can be easily combined with Western naturopathy or even scientifically oriented conventional medicine.

## AYURVEDA: HOW TO LEAD A HEALTHY LIFE

I decided to meet with Syal Kumar, a doctor trained in Western as well as traditional Indian medicine. Kumar came from a family dynasty of Ayurvedic physicians in Kerala, one of the birthplaces of Ayurveda. It was especially important to him that Ayurveda was understood and used as a healing method, not as an exotic wellness program. We began a discussion on what could be achieved with Ayurveda in Germany, especially in combination with Western medicine. Finally, my plans were made: I would bring him to the hospital in Essen. We thought about how we could integrate the Ayurvedic approach to therapy and garner a valuable collection of scientific data at the same time. As a first step, we bought an Indian treatment couch made of wood for oil treatments, an important part of this healing method.

In 2006, many Germans had already heard of Ayurveda, but patients had mainly images of palm-lined beaches and Shirodhara in their heads when we suggested an Ayurvedic treatment to them. In fact, Ayurveda is a complete system of diagnosis and therapies. In my opinion, it is the traditional healing method with the greatest body of practical knowledge and the most extensive collection of treatment details in the world. Records of European Medieval healing methods have—with a few exceptions, such as the works of Hildegard von Bingen—not survived. Traditional Chinese Medicine was largely revived in the twentieth century through state-controlled measures and programmatic politics initiated by Mao Zedong, since the huge country could not be supplied with Western medicine comprehensively, and because there was a desire to market parts of the healing system, especially acupuncture, successfully in the West.[1]

Ayurveda, on the other hand, has been practiced continuously for more than two thousand years. Accordingly, this healing tradition is an equal to modern medicine, recognized by the Indian government and bordering South Asian nations. Every year, hundreds of millions of people in South Asia are treated primarily with Ayurveda—while conventional medicine is only used in emergency cases.

By now, Ayurveda is recognized as a medicinal science by the WHO as well. In India itself, there are more than 400,000 registered Ayurvedic doctors and more than 250 tertiary institutions that offer an extensive training in Ayurveda, which lasts five to eight years. Ayurvedic physicians work at more than 2,500 hospitals and 15,000 outpatient clinics. This shows that in its country of origin, Ayurveda is anything but a wellness treatment.

At the center of Ayurveda stands the teachings of a healthy life—*ayus* meaning "life," and *veda* meaning "the knowledge." Their roots are anchored in the Vedas, the holy Indian texts that incorporate physical, psychological, and spiritual aspects of healing. In India, Ayurveda is also a reverence to the gods. After all, according to tradition, the creator god Brahma personally gifted this knowledge to humans.

Symptoms can be treated in numerous ways in Ayurveda, depending on the patient's type. That the combination of body type, physical appearance, and behavior says something about the predisposition for certain diseases is also recognized in German naturopathy. In Ayurveda these factors are taken into consideration to choose the right therapies for each individual. You have probably already heard about the *doshas*: the combination of body type, skin, and hair, as well as the characteristics of numerous other physical traits that make up the three basic types in Indian medicine—*vata*, *pitta*, and *kapha*. But forget about the *dosha* tests you may have seen in magazines, cookbooks, or on the internet. All people are mixed types, and what constitution and individuality is present exactly can only be determined with professional experience.

In Sanskrit, the language in which the Ayurvedic texts (some that date back two thousand years) are written, the word "constitution" is called *prakrti* ("nature"). Constitution is inherent and doesn't change, unlike the symptoms that it produces as a result of stimuli and stresses. These symptoms are called *vikrti* ("disturbances"), and it's these disturbances that are being treated. Similar to the concepts of Chinese medicine, the *doshas* also express opposite poles of characteristics: *vata* symbolizes wind and movement, the airy. This can either be interpreted as ease or as being under too much stress ("being rattled"). *Pitta* symbolizes temperature, energy, and metabolism. Change, in other words, that is caused by fire. *Kapha* means "construction" and "mass" and is found in water and earth.

## AYURVEDA THINKS IN CHARACTERISTICS

I would like to demonstrate here how complex the structure of Ayurveda is. The content, form, and direction of movement of a disruption are always analyzed and treated in conjunction with one another. The *doshas* exemplify principles that illustrate the three major areas of reaction patterns in a simplified manner. With their help, we as doctors keep track of the complexity of events in the body and the psyche. But the *dosha* theory can by no means explain all medical details. It would be too simplistic to divide all people and all diseases into only three groups. "The *doshas* are like primary colors," explains Elmar Stapelfeldt, an Indologist and expert on Ayurveda who counsels many patients at the Immanuel Hospital in Berlin: "By using different mixing ratios, millions of colors are described and explained as patient histories."

To describe the *doshas* more precisely, they are each allocated seven characteristics, the *gunas*. An arthrosis in the shoulder joint, for example, is attributed to an excess of *gunas* (dryness) and thus ascribed to the *vata* area. In Western medicine we diagnose a loss of synovial fluid and a painful constriction of the joint cavity coupled with a roughening of the cartilage layer—also a kind of dryness.

Western medicine is guided by a molecular biological model of the body—and analyzes enzymes, hormones, neurotransmitters, genes, or pathogens. That's why it has developed into a highly specialized science that tries, on the micro level, to change, supplement, or disable some of these biological substances according to the lock-and-key model. Ayurveda, on the other hand, thinks in characteristics. "Movement," the main characteristic of *vata*, fosters a milieu that generates stress symptoms, tension, indigestion, and concentration disorders. In the long run, "sour" (*pitta*) leads to inflammations whereas "sweet" (*kapha*) carries obesity and the danger of diabetes with it.

An essential instrument for influencing an imbalance of the *doshas*, and thus the symptoms of diseases, is nutrition. The power of digesting food is seen as the center of the body. This includes all substances and functions that dissemble the food, transform, and excrete it. Imagine a stove at the center of your body that needs a lot of energy to process a meal. That's why we become tired after eating. The more indigestible things we eat—the heavier, more compact, and colder a meal is—the more energy we use, and this energy is then lacking in other areas of the body.

# The Ayurvedic Treatment of Arthrosis

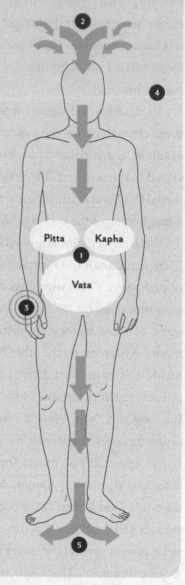

**1 Understanding the Sickness**
According to the teachings of Ayurveda, every human being contains a balance of three *doshas*, or constitutional types: vata, pitta, kapha. If one of the doshas is excessively dominant, symptoms of a disease develop. The aim of Ayurvedic treatment is to reinstate a balance of the constitutional types.

**2 Sickening Factors**
Poor diet, physical stress, trauma, worries, anxieties, stress, suppression of bodily needs

**3 Symptoms**
Pain, inflammations, degradation of cartilage, and restriction of movement are typical symptoms of *vata*.

**4 Diagnosis**
By observing the tongue, eyes, physique, urine, feces, heart rate, palpating, auscultation, as well as using modern diagnostics: laboratory and imaging methods

**5 Therapy**
Reducing the *vata* through excretion (e.g., purging, sweat baths), manual therapies (e.g., massages), treatment with medications (e.g., nose oil, medicinal herbs), diet, behavioral modifications (e.g., daily-, sleep-, and eating rhythms)

Internal heat is central in Indian medicine. Internal heat is fueled by warming soups, ginger tea, and spices. In Ayurveda, spices are an everyday component of a healthy life. They are meant to stimulate the *agni*, the "digestive fire." Modern nutritional science focuses on the ingredients of food and places little importance on how meals are consumed and processed within the body. But in Ayurveda the physician diagnoses the condition of the *agni* as a key factor. It can be weak, slow, and sluggish (*mandagni*), a sign of the *kapha dosha*; this leads to burping or bloating. An irregular *agni* (*vishamagni*) changes often, fitting the "animated" *vata* type. In *pitta* people, the *agni* is often "too sharp, penetrating" (*tikshnagni*). People of this type are often hungry, suffer from acid reflux, and don't put on weight, no matter how much they eat.

Supporting the *agni* is the first and most important step of Ayurvedic nutritional therapy. This first step is easy to implement and maintain and is quite effective. In the second step, the individual dosha is taken into account for specific recommendations—such as eating less wheat, avoiding certain kinds of vegetables or spices or, on the contrary, using larger quantities of them.

Finally, there is the *mala*, which we would translate as "by-products and wastes." Generally, *mala* denotes all substances that do not belong in the body, i.e., environmental toxins, unhealthy foods, tobacco, alcohol, and particularly metabolites that have not been broken down. In Ayurveda these substances are called "sticky"—they aren't easy to get rid of. When you try to excrete them, you harm tissue that occurs naturally in the body—as though you were trying to squeeze juice from unripe fruit. It is necessary to stimulate the metabolism first in order to transfer the *mala* into a state in which it can be excreted. This is achieved by fasting or through eating light, warm meals. According to Ayurveda, animal proteins contained in meat and cheese (especially mold cheese) as well as cold foods are generally hard to digest.

Just as Ayurvedic medicine focuses not on individual substances but on complex relationships between characteristics, it also doesn't take an interest in individual cells or organs, but in entire tissues. They permeate the whole body and symptoms manifest themselves in them. An important term in this is the *rasa*, the nutritive fluid. It contains the nutrients that are distributed to all tissues via the blood. *Rasa* is a force that also includes mental and immunologic bodily defenses. Healing oils that are often massaged into the skin are involved in its regeneration. Fatty acids also ensure that the plant-based components are able to penetrate the connective tissue better.

It's not always easy for patients to think in processes and characteristics in this manner, especially since it can contradict our general idea about what is "healthy." There are no healthy or unhealthy foodstuffs in Ayurveda, only suitable or unsuitable ones. An orange, rich in vitamin C, may be healthy according to Western thinking, but is wrong for a *pitta* type. The same goes for pickled vegetables, i.e., vegetables that have been preserved by malolactic fermentation or immersion in vinegar and that are considered a health food in the West because of their lactobacilli content.

Patients quickly notice how pleasant changing their dietary habits is. Then they are delighted to find that they not only feel better with having a warm lunch, which they had hitherto denied themselves, but that they also tend to lose weight—because the "digestive fire" is unburdened by it. Many value Ayurvedic dietary therapy also because it's easy to integrate into their daily routine.

Even the initial experiences with food showed that Ayurveda has an immense potential. We recommended Ayurvedic treatment to patients who didn't achieve sufficient successes despite our extensive range of naturopathic therapies—often with surprisingly positive results.

## MY FIRST JOURNEY TO INDIA

In 2007, I decided to go to India for the first time in order to get to know the country and the people, but of course also Ayurveda, first-hand. It was love at first sight. The colors, the diversity of people, the spices, the odors—people who have never driven through an Indian city before wonder where this zest for life and joy come from, especially as the conditions seem more than exhausting and difficult to a German. But I'll never forget how I was walking through Frankfurt airport after landing in Germany, noticing a completely different kind of stress, and I thought I sensed a lot of tension or even grief in people. Afterward, I asked myself again and again how such an enormous discrepancy between objective standards of living and the subjective enjoyment of life can occur.

After several days of meditation in an ashram, my wife and I ventured to Kerala to explore Ayurveda on-site. We flew to Kochi, an ancient spice trading center. It was the most horrible flight of my life and it made me significantly more religious. A beautiful hotel from colonial times—the Bolgatty Palace—distracted us from it after we landed. Syal Kumar, who was on home leave in Kerala at the time, talked to a local physician about our respective Ayurvedic treatments—it was the only way I could get a direct impression.

I was looking forward to the therapy, and expected relaxation from it. But things turned out differently. After the third day with a special diet and different oil treatments, which lasted one and a half hours each, I experienced a tiredness I had never felt before—as if somebody had unplugged me. I hadn't expected that. I also noted this very strong effect during subsequent Ayurvedic therapies such as Shirodhara, the pouring of liquids over the forehead, or the Abhyanga, the full-body massage. It manifested itself mainly in the form of a great need for sleep. One time, colleagues in Berlin gave me a Shirodhara treatment as a birthday gift. I had made the appointment for 2 to 3 p.m. and thought that this would be a good way to refresh myself before the subsequent meetings. But after the Shirodhara treatment there was no way that I could go through any type of activity—I was so tired that I had to cancel the meetings and lie down in bed at home. But the following day I felt splendid. I know of no other method that can alleviate great stress in such a manner.

By now studies have proven the profound effect Shirodhara has on relieving stress and anxiety. So far, we are unable to explain why that is so. Maybe reflexive neuroplexus play a part in it, because they are stimulated in a very special way by the continuous application of the oil. There is a reason, after all, for why the forehead area in its symbolism is important in Ayurveda, just as in yoga. It is the "third eye," a sign of blessing, that can be found in Hindu temples. According to Indian tradition, the forehead *chakra* is of eminent importance for the human consciousness.

But most of all, I had experienced both during Shirodhara and the full-body massage of Abhyanga a certain disorientation that is induced in a therapeutic manner that then slows down the constant flow of thoughts. In a classic massage, we can always tell where the hand of the massage therapist is at any given moment. But when we are massaged by two people, i.e., by four hands (sometimes there are even more people involved in the oil treatments), this becomes impossible after only a few minutes. You have to submit to the treatment, have to let go. In addition, there is the effect the medicinal oil has. The process in Shirodhara is similar: The gentle flow of oil that spreads over the entire forehead (the eyes are protected by a blindfold) is applied continuously for up to forty minutes. This unusual experience ultimately leads to a kind of transposition, to a changed perception of the body.

Why I became so particularly tired during these treatments every time is also related to my constitution. People with a very tight schedule and great intellectual pressure to concentrate often show a *vata* tendency. According to Ayurveda, too many elements of motion are active in these cases. Shirodhara and Abhyanga slow down the over-stimulated senses substantially to induce recreation. But after such therapies, the exhaustion is felt much more strongly, because *vata* types tend to ignore their need for rest (and instead drink an espresso to counteract the fatigue).

Back to Kerala. Once my wife and I had recovered somewhat from the flight, we set out to visit Ayurvedic hospitals in the following days. It was impressive. I realized that in India, Ayurveda is used to treat very serious, very severe illnesses. One hospital was close to one of the most accident-prone motorways in the state. After acute care was administered, many of the crash victims were also treated with Ayurveda, just like paraplegic patients with neurological diseases like Parkinson's or multiple sclerosis. It was clear that everyone was satisfied. The doctors seemed professional, well-trained, and legitimate. They described and explained the treatments to us. It seemed as though Ayurvedic therapy with plant-based drugs was of particularly great value in especially severe diseases.

## INDIA'S RICH PHARMACY OF HERBS AND SPICES

As a naturopath, I was naturally familiar with phytotherapy, the use of medicinal plants. I value European herbal medicine, but I am aware of its limitations. But Ayurveda uses a special technique of drug therapy that makes it more effective than its European counterpart. It involves two things: On one hand, India's herbal pharmacy is significantly richer than our European one, because more medicinal plants grow in the local climate. Close to one thousand different herbs are generally utilized in Ayurvedic pharmacies. On the other hand, however, it's not individual substances that are administered in a maximum dosage, but sometimes up to fifty different components are mixed in various proportions and then administered for therapy in this individualized composition. The principle behind this is evident and resembles that of Chinese phytotherapy: One picks out herbs and plants that in combination fortify the desired effect, but that have different side effects. That's why these do not add up but stay underneath the perceptional threshold.

This is a smart principle, but also one of the challenges in bringing Ayurveda to the Western world. Our pharmacology eliminated these kinds of mixtures of substances for the most part in the 1980s, when regulations made it mandatory to identify the most essential agent in each drug and to describe its mechanism of action in a plant monograph. Ever since then, the majority of plant-based drugs have disappeared from the market, because the manufacturers were no longer able to finance elaborate studies or because the mechanism of action wasn't simply based on one individual substance. Only a few mixtures whose harmlessness had been proven through decades of use survived this legal change.

Today, phytopharmacology is predominantly "rational": One identifies the substance to which the effect is ascribed. After a series of laboratory testing, experiments on animals and dose-response studies on humans, the drug with the designated main substance—and only this drug—is approved for therapeutic use. It's evident that individualized mixtures of substances containing up to fifty individual substances combined in a different way for each patient could never conform to our standards.

But if Ayurvedic medicaments weren't considered drugs but rather a nutritional supplement and were then imported, as it is often the case in both the United States and Germany, we would face the problem of insufficient quality- and safety control of the extracts. This can have undesired, even dangerous effects on the patients treated with them. But do we really want to deny the chance to recover the great treasures of Ayurvedic pharmacology simply because they don't comply with our regulations? This would be a great shame, because the successful healings that I have observed until now by far exceed that which can be explained with the placebo effect or spontaneous recovery.

The institutions concerned with the regulation of drugs and therapeutic devices would be well advised to convene with the Indian government (or the Chinese authorities) in a constructive manner in order to make these therapeutic options available to the world. A special registration process for Ayurvedic compounds would be the most sensible solution, because ultimately, they cannot be classified as either food or drugs but are somewhere in the middle.

It should also be noted that phytopharmaceuticals, or "multitarget" pharmacology, are much more adapted to the biology of the human body than the mono-target approach that we cultivate in Western pharmacology. Though Western pharmacology may be very successful in addressing some diseases, we need to acknowledge that the side effects of drugs have grown to such a magnitude that they themselves are one of the most common causes of deaths.[2] Furthermore, they are the reason many patients don't take their medication as prescribed—in some drugs the lack of compliance reaches between 60 and 70 percent.[3]

When I became head of the naturopathic department at the Immanuel Hospital in Berlin two years after my first trip to India, it was my goal to integrate Ayurveda as one of the central pillars there. Fortunately, Christian Kessler, a young internist and Indologist who had attained a great reputation with his knowledge of Ayurveda, was already employed at the Charité. We agreed that it was time to base Ayurveda on solid scientific research and integrate it into treatments. Together with Claudia Witt, who held an endowed professorship for Complementary Medicine at the Charité at the time (today she teaches at the University of Zurich), we conceptualized an extensive study designed to examine the effectiveness of Ayurveda. We got in touch with the European Academy for Ayurveda in Birstein, Germany, whose medical superintendent S. N. Gupta is one of the most internationally renowned experts on Ayurveda, but also with Antonio Morandi at the Center for Ayurveda in Milan, and Ludwig Kronpaß in Bavaria.

## ILLNESSES THAT CAN BE TREATED WITH AYURVEDA

The longer I researched Ayurveda, the more I realized what could be the most important indicators for this Indian art of healing in Europe:

1. Diabetes. There are many interesting plant-based substances that have already been proven to lower blood sugar levels, such as the bitter melon or the herbal mixture Triphala.[4]
2. Neurological diseases. Not only was I able to observe the successful treatment of neurological diseases in Kerala, but also, one of the world's leading experts on Parkinson's disease, Horst Przuntek, has dedicated himself to Ayurveda after leaving his position as medical director of the University Hospitals of the Ruhr-University of Bochum. He founded a Department for Neurology and Ayurveda at the Protestant Hospital in Hattingen and since then has been treating patients with multiple sclerosis, Parkinson's, and other neurodegenerative diseases.

     Early on, Przuntek pointed out that the Ayurvedic treatment of patients with Parkinson's happened primarily via the olfactory sense (by inunction with nose oil) and the intestine (through the cleansing ritual Panchakarma and diet). Possibly, these treatments target the areas that are considered the point of origin for Parkinson's according to most recent scientific findings—the olfactory brain on one hand and the microbiome on the other.[5] Fascinating. It seems as though Ayurveda already knew two thousand years ago what we are only now discovering through highly technologized molecular biological analyses.

3. Rheumatism and arthrosis. In 2011, the American rheumatologist Daniel Furst, together with our close Indian cooperation partner Ram Manohar, presented a study comparing Ayurvedic treatment of rheumatism and arthrosis to the conventional Western treatment using the antirheumatic agent Methotrexate. They were able to show that the treatments were similarly successful.[6]

4. Bowel diseases. And finally, Ayurveda is also successful in treating bowel diseases. In addition to having Christian Kessler at our hospital, we were able to bring Elmar Stapelfeldt as well. Stapelfeldt has expanded the treatment focus of nutritional therapy. Even with naturopathy it's difficult to treat common disorders like an irritable colon or the ever-increasing number of food intolerances. Therefore, it has been even more surprising to see how the simple therapeutic principles of Ayurveda can help—often without avoiding the apparently responsible foods.

To me, these indicators seemed the most important argument for implementing Ayurveda in medicine. But in principle, every disease can be addressed with the multimodal treatment principle. The aim of our newly founded Department for Ayurveda was to conduct a meaningful study on the effectiveness of Ayurveda therapy in a common chronic disease. We decided on arthrosis. After many phone calls, and with the support of several Indian Ayurvedic physicians, we ulti-mately succeeded in getting the Indian embassy in Berlin on board.

And so we convened in my office at the Immanuel Hospital in Ber-lin one afternoon and formulated the following goal: A study on the efficiency of traditional multimodal Ayurveda in comparison to the best Western conventional medicine in treating arthrosis of the knees. The Indian ambassador was willing to support us, but he also made it clear that we would have to present our project in Delhi in person. He initiated all the necessary steps.

## A RESEARCH COOPERATION WITH INDIA

I traveled to Delhi with Mark Rosenberg from the European Academy for Ayurveda. I had prepared a presentation and a lecture that was meant to clarify how important it was to conduct a clinical study on the impact of Ayurveda in order to give this Indian art of healing the recognition it deserved in the West—provided we saw good results. We were unsure whether it would be possible to obtain the initial re-search funding outside India for such a study.

At the Federal Ministry of Health, we were met by Jalaja Devi, the state secretary for Ayurveda. When we entered the room, we received skeptical looks from roughly a dozen employees of the ministry. After a few introductory remarks, Mark Rosenberg told them that Ayurveda was enjoying growing popularity in Germany. After that, I described the planned concept of our study, and tried to explain how much I wished that Ayurveda would open itself up to clinical science. Subse-quently, we were asked many critical questions that all essentially re-volved around the issue of whether we would be able to meet the requirements of Ayurveda. We also spoke about the costs for the study that were due to the great expenses for staff.

Over and over, we were asked why the German government wasn't funding such a study. I replied that obtaining German research funding for traditional Indian medicine was a completely futile endeavor at the moment since we would first have to prove that Ayurveda was a therapy that had to be taken seriously. Only when this initial step had been taken with one or two good studies could there be possibilities for German funding of future studies. Finally, Jalaja Devi knocked on the table and the room fell silent. After a short query about whether the Charité belonged to Humboldt University, she explained to the group that this is where the highest standard of Indology outside of the country, maybe even better than in India itself, was taught. This could also be the case for Ayurveda now. Nobody disagreed with her, two assistants entered with contracts, and we posed for a group photo. When Mark Rosenberg and I found ourselves back outside the Ministry of Health, blinking in the spring sun, we couldn't believe it—we had managed to obtain the financial foundation for the first large-scale clinical study on Ayurveda in the Western world.

**PATIENT HISTORY**

## Arthrosis
*Medicinal Herbs Instead of Artificial Joints*

The pain had to be almost unbearable, but the patient, an engineer in her early sixties, kept a straight face. She had severe arthrosis of the knee joints, the wrists, and the ankles. In regular intervals, the pain returned with such intensity that she was unable to work, use a computer, or take the stairs. She agreed to have a surgery to remove calcification in her right middle finger. It achieved nothing. Was she supposed to keep taking more and more pain medication and eventually damage her kidneys because of it? The patient had seen a television report on naturopathic alternatives and came to see us.

She was being treated by Christian Kessler, our expert on medical Ayurveda. She started to take turmeric (Indian saffron) and incense as nutritional supplements—which are working well for her. Both substances have an anti-inflammatory effect and cause cells to regenerate. The metabolism and digestion are stimulated. Indian phytotherapy, however, does not rely on merely one individual agent, but on a mixture of active agents. That's why one shouldn't take turmeric isolated in a pill or a powder. Instead, it should be ingested in the form of curry. But to achieve a positive effect it's necessary to use one teaspoon of pure turmeric powder (in combination with black pepper) every day.

The patient was overweight, which also put strain on her joints. Her blood pressure was elevated, and she was taking a beta blocker for that. When she came to the clinic for the first time, she weighed 181 lbs. at a height of 5'6". Within one year she lost 8.8 lbs. by switching to an Ayurvedic-vegetarian diet. She has been able to cut out the beta blockers and her blood pressure is back to normal. She is only allowed to lose weight slowly so that the body can adapt and doesn't "strike back" with a yo-yo effect. What did the patient eat? Lots of vegetables, usually in the form of soups, chutneys, or curries, prepared at warm temperatures. For the most part, she left out anything that fostered inflammations in her body: wheat, sugar, alcohol, meat.

In addition to all this, the patient started practicing yoga. Strengthening the muscles, connective tissues, and the spine helps the joints. To fortify this effect, my colleague Kessler and his team gave the patient an Ayurvedic massage with medicinal oils, such as a warm carrier oil like sesame combined with cilantro, cumin, and myrrh, once a week over the course of two months. After each massage she had a sweat bath. This causes the pores to open and enables the oils to penetrate deeper into the tissue. Today the patient is completely free of symptoms.

## AYURVEDA: BOTH PREVENTION AND THERAPY

Ayurveda is the essence of a holistic healing system. It is concerned with four major areas:

1. Prevention, i.e., the avoidance of causes and the strengthening of patients' self-efficacy.
2. Balancing methods, i.e., nutritional, organizational, and phyto-therapeutic.
3. Channeling methods—via the intestine, the blood, or the nose—i.e., douches, enemas, or nasal applications. This also includes therapeutic vomiting, the use of leeches, and bloodletting. External excretions are stimulated by oil massages, Scotch hose treatments, sweat baths, rice poultices, or intensive manual therapies. In the Ayurvedic concept, surgery is also important and categorized as a channeling procedure.
4. Another independent area is spirituality. Ayurveda without spirituality, without a direct connection to meditation and yoga, is unimaginable. That is another asset, because numerous studies have proven that religious or spiritual entrenchment is accompanied by a better prognosis and better chances of recovery.[7, 8, 9]

In 2011, the Indian government established a database called
DHARA (dharaonline.org), in which studies and reports of healing
are collected and the results of earlier studies are documented.
Ayurveda is not a simple healing model but a highly complex one. One
also can't allege that it is possible to get rich from it quickly. It's an
elaborate therapy, from the pharmacological production of the medications to the intensive personal care of the treatments.

This may pose a challenge in the future. When the number of
studies on the positive effects of Ayurveda grow, our healthcare system will have to discuss whether the costs for Ayurvedic treatments
will be absorbed by health insurance companies, and if there are
cheaper alternatives (even if these cheaper alternatives may be subject
to more side effects). For now, Ayurvedic therapies have to be paid for
out of one's own pocket—with one exception: Since our department
for Ayurvedic medicine in Berlin is part of the Charité's university
hospital outpatient clinic, patients with public health insurance can
use the opportunity to have Ayurvedic nutrition counseling.

Regarding the cleanliness of medicinal plants and phytotherapeu-
tic preparations, I recommend buying Ayurvedic medicines and preparations only in pharmacies that carry out purity controls. Still, to be
honest, it's possible that even legitimate Indian manufacturers of
medications deliver batches of heavily contaminated medication. This
is due to the *rasa shastra*, a branch of Indian pharmacology in which
small doses of heavy metals such as lead and mercury are used for
therapeutic measures. In keeping with our Western knowledge, such a
use cannot be approved of by any means.

## THE PRINCIPLES OF AYURVEDA ARE UNIVERSAL

According to the principle of hormesis, it's theoretically not to be ruled out that this negative opinion may be revised at some point, because even toxic substances in small doses can have positive effects. But that is pure speculation. At the moment it must be assumed that the administration of even small amounts of heavy metals can cause severe damage. What's problematic is that some manufacturers aren't separating the production areas and as a result, volatile mercury contaminates other medications. Additionally, the soil and the air in India (as in China) are heavily polluted by environmental toxins.

We advise our patients to use selected manufacturers with very strict controls. Beyond that, Christian Kessler and Elmar Stapelfeldt have developed concepts for substitution plant-based Indian medications based on a selection of foods and European spices. It's also conceivable to choose selected European medicinal plants according to the teachings and the standards of Ayurveda in some recipes—because the principles of Ayurveda are universal. They can be adjusted for every form of nutrition and drug administration. It might even be more sensible for people of European origin to use European foods and plants, since our genetic code and our constitution are adapted to them. This would reinforce the recommendation to eat seasonally and locally (albeit with the disadvantage of not utilizing the potential and the ancient knowledge of Ayurveda to the fullest extent).

Ayurveda is a multimodal treatment method and medicinal system with an abundance of therapeutic details and a distinct focus on individualization that maximizes therapeutic success. Additionally, it possesses highly developed methods of pulse and tongue diagnosis.

We can all feel our heart rate in our chest and in our pulse. When we're excited our hearts jump or race. There are countless proverbs that point out this experience of our heart. This is significantly different from all the other organs of the human body that do their work without us being able to feel it. We don't notice our liver detoxing or our kidney producing urine, but we do feel our heart pumping blood into our lungs and limbs.

In Ayurveda as well as in Traditional Chinese Medicine the art of feeling the pulse plays a rather essential role. Not only is the speed of the pulse (pulse rate) evaluated, but also how voluminous, tense, soft, or hard the pulse feels. The wealth of knowledge on pulse diagnosis is astonishingly great, but until now, science has been unable to explain unambiguously how intricately these categories are actually connected to tangible diseases. It's very easy to detect the fact that the pulse rate is subject to change for yourself. If you feel your pulse at the same time every day for several weeks, you'll find out relatively quickly that it does indeed feel weaker or stronger some days, that it may at times seem tense or jumping. With some practice it won't be hard to notice how this actually does relate to the condition of the body's strength and health.

I for one am convinced that we shouldn't underestimate the significance of this historically proven phenomenology despite all the euphoria for the rapid progress in epigenetics and molecular biology. It should be our goal to conserve the old—on a scientific basis—and apply it as part of modern concepts.

## ACUPUNCTURE: SUCCESSFUL IN TREATING PAIN

Traditional Chinese Medicine encompasses a number of different therapeutic methods: diet, phytomedicine, massage (*tuina*), meditative movement patterns like qigong and tai chi. In the West, it's predominantly acupuncture (from the Latin *acus* meaning "needle," and *pungere* meaning "to jab") that has prevailed, which doesn't actually play an essential part in China itself. But since it's the method whose complexity was most easily reduced to Western understanding, it has firmly situated itself in medicine and is now employed by many European physicians. It is that method of complementary medicine that has been researched in the best and most extensive manner.

The starting point for this development was President Richard Nixon's state visit to China in 1972. An accompanying reporter from the *New York Times*, James Reston, had to undergo an appendectomy there. He was subsequently treated with nothing but acupuncture and was able to avoid pain medication completely, an experience he described enthusiastically. His reportage made its way around the globe and awoke the international interest in acupuncture. By now we know that acupuncture can indeed be an excellent way to treat pain.

The largest worldwide studies on acupuncture were conducted in Germany. Thousands of patients with different pain disorders were treated with acupuncture in precisely predetermined settings at the Charité Hospital and the Ruhr-University in Bochum. The effect was then compared in sophisticated clinical studies—to pain medication, but also to feigned acupuncture (where, unnoticed by the patients, the needle was not inserted), or to minimal acupuncture (where the needle penetrated the skin, but not at the traditional acupuncture points). This was designed to clarify whether the pricking with needles didn't simply have a great placebo effect.

The results of the studies proved two things very clearly: First, that acupuncture relieves pain very well in many pain disorders, for example in chronic lumbar back pains, neck pain, shoulder pain, but also in pain caused by arthrosis, headaches, and migraines, or a neuropathy (disorders of the nervous system). Second, that the effect consists of

two components, a specific effect that is actually achieved by the precise pricking at the traditional acupuncture points, and the psychological effect of the treatment situation, the ritual and the penetration
of the skin wherein the traditional acupuncture points are no longer
relevant.[10, 11, 12, 13] The results were so convincing, particularly where
back pain and arthrosis of the knees were concerned, that ever since
then, the costs for acupuncture treatment have been absorbed by
health insurance companies in these cases.

Still, the studies were unable to explain how and why acupuncture
is effective. That acupuncture also achieves effects when the traditional
points aren't stimulated was taken as evidence by critics that it's just a
placebo therapy after all. The supporters pointed out the overall excellent treatment successes. For example, supplementary acupuncture
was compared to the standard treatment by GPs and orthopedists—
patients who had received acupuncture were doing significantly better.
And in my opinion, that's what counts first and foremost.

The studies taught us doctors that things can't be simplified too
much. Part of the effect of acupuncture is created by trust in the therapist, by the atmosphere of care and calm in the treatment situation—
just as it is in every doctor-patient relationship. Another part is created
by the pricking of the needle itself. This can have an effect on all the
organs in the body. Every student of medicine knows the so-called
Head's zones, skin areas each body possesses. Each of these zones is
supplied by a nerve. This nerve enters the spinal marrow at the spine
and sends nerve signals to the brain. Since that's where nerve signals
from the inner organs also arrive, there is a direct contact between our
outer skin nerves and the internal nerves of the organs and the connective tissue. That's why the stimulus of an acupuncture needle can
cause an effect in the deeper layers of the connective tissue and even
in the inner organs. The Head's zones are broader than the narrow

meridians described by Traditional Chinese Medicine. So, it is not surprising that the acupuncture needle doesn't have to be placed accurate to the millimeter to have an effect.

Beyond that, however, there are also very precise, point-specific effects. According to the data derived from the largest study on acupuncture so far, the Acupuncture Trialists' Collaboration with more than twenty thousand subjects, this point-specific effect constitutes about a third of the overall effect.[14] To understand this, we don't necessarily have to accept meridians or *chi* as a concept. There are enough special trigger points or receptors in our fasciae on an anatomic basis that are very important for pain to develop and that show very strong consistency with the traditional acupuncture points.

It would be interesting to know how people in ancient China came to this realization roughly three thousand years ago. The traditional concept of acupuncture is impressive with the sophistication of its detailed knowledge and its figurative language. It assumes that the energy necessary for life (*qi*) flows through the body along specific pathways (meridians). When the flow of energy is disrupted, for example by environmental influences like cold, warmth, air drafts, or incorrect diet, emotional strain, and overexertion, physical symptoms can develop. The flow of energy can be influenced in a therapeutic manner at more than seven hundred specific points (acupuncture points) through pressure (acupressure), warmth (moxibustion), or the jabbing with a needle (acupuncture).

Even though acupuncture's specific mechanism of action has not yet been explained fully from a Western point of view, certain aspects are known. What has been observed are the increased release of pain-relieving endorphins, neurotransmitters, and tissue hormones which are conducive to relaxation. Furthermore, stimuli that have an effect inside the body are applied via the skin areas—just like a disease of the gallbladder can cause pain in the right shoulder blade, a classic phenomenon of internal medicine. That's why acupuncture has been able to gain a foothold particularly in pain therapy.

But acupuncture can also be effective in the treatment of other diseases. In a methodologically sophisticated study, my colleague Benno Brinkhaus at the Charité Hospital randomly divided more than 420 patients with severe hay fever (seasonal allergic rhinitis) into three groups: The first received commonly used antihistaminic drugs if needed, the second received mock-acupuncture, and the third received point-specific acupuncture. All of the patients were allowed to take antihistamines as emergency medication in case their symptoms were too grave. Ultimately the group that received traditional acupuncture did significantly better in comparison, and the effect was noticeable even one year later. This study, funded by the German Research Foundation, is further proof for the fact that acupuncture mustn't be dismissed as a pseudo-therapy.[15]

Acupuncture can also serve well as a supplementary cancer treatment. It relieves nausea and vomiting and even nerve disorders caused by chemotherapy. The fatigue from which cancer patients suffer, and which is usually difficult to treat, can be alleviated and treated with acupuncture.[16]

In China the schism between "modern medicine" and "traditional medicine" doesn't exist. Since 1982, Traditional Chinese Medicine (TCM) has been officially recognized next to Western medicine. All major specialist disciplines can be found at the hospital of the renowned Sun Yat-Sen University in the metropolitan city of Guangzhou, from gastroenterology to rheumatology; on every floor there is one completely conventional and one integrative department, in which nutritional therapy, acupuncture, and medicinal herbs are used as supplementary treatments. When I visited the hospital, I immediately noticed the large research building next to the hospital. In China, it's quite commonplace for the TCM physicians working at the hospital to conduct scientific work in some form or other as well. This gives cause to hope that this is where a scientifically grounded medicine is making its way.

## THE HEALING POWER OF PLANTS

The biggest potential of TCM lies in its herbal medicine. The 5,600 officinal (from the Latin *officina*, meaning "workshop" or "pharmacy") components of Chinese pharmacology include medicinal plants and mineral substances as well as mushrooms and products of animal origin. A selection of roughly 500 plants is used particularly often, but only a few of these are known in the West (these are plants such as ginseng, ginkgo, Japanese mint, rhubarb, or licorice). The origins of China's pharmacotherapy are ascribed to the mythological figure of Shennong ("God Farmer"). It is said that he was testing plants for their potential powers as early as the third century BC. The script *Wushi'er Bingfang, Recipes for Fifty-Two Ailments*, written in the third century BC, copied onto sheets of silk, and found as a burial object in Mawangdui, is the first written compendium.

There are many questions about the safety and quality of Chinese medicine. Imports from China may be contaminated, sometimes even counterfeit. When the bales of exotic dried herbs arrive, the identity and purity of the substances they contain ought to be tested. Unknown interactions are particularly problematic, especially in patients suffering from chronic diseases who take multiple medications at the same time. Beyond that, it's possible that some substances have an additional hormone-like effect. That's why a therapy with Chinese medicine requires a lot of knowledge and experience as well as a continuous monitoring of its effects.

But this shouldn't deter us from further research and application of this enormous therapeutic potential. If such interactions are considered and examined further, if the imports are controlled and the medicinal plants are grown locally (as was done in an experiment in Bavaria), and finally, if the art of the correct application is mastered, Chinese pharmacotherapy, similar to Ayurveda, is greatly suitable in a combination with Western therapies in integrative medicine.

In all the major traditional healing arts around the world, plants—in the form of compresses, teas, spices, or foods—occupy center stage. I have already mentioned this for Ayurveda and in Traditional Chinese Medicine. But it should be assumed that the therapeutic use of medicinal plants is as old as humanity itself. Plants, animals, and humans have evolved in reciprocal adaptation. Through evolution, a lavish abundance of substances developed over the course of millions of years, among them those that were, and still are, important for the survival of the plants: These phytochemicals serve to lure insects or other animals so that pollination or dissemination of the plant is ensured—they lend the plant a certain color or create aromatic oils. Other phytochemicals are bitter constituents or the poison digitalis—they ward off predators or microbes. Some of these substances are so potent that the plants merely develop them in harmless preliminary stages and only transform them into the poisonous final product that has a much stronger effect in case of an emergency, for example when a larva bites into a leaf.

It's mainly these substances—next to nutritional components such as carbohydrates, proteins, and oils—that are responsible for the healing potential. Generally, they are bitter, spicy, or otherwise unpleasant. Humans probably followed their instincts when they resorted to using them in certain circumstances, like in case of a fever. Animals can be observed to ingest special plants that wouldn't normally be part of their diet when they are ill. Bugs, for example, start eating medicinally effective plants when they are infested by parasites. When healthy, they would avoid this "medicine."[17] The "self-medication" of animals by changing their feeding behavior has by now become its own, young branch of research in biology, called zoopharmacognosy. Our herbal medicine (phytotherapy) can learn a lot by observing it. For instance, African elephants search for borages before giving birth. These have a labor-inducing effect, and by now extracts of these plants are used in Kenya by pregnant women when they give birth.[18]

The body is able to detoxicate small amounts of toxic substances in the intestine or in the liver. Sometimes it's enough to give the plant a little time and to imitate nature: The hot mustard oils derived from crucifers such as broccoli or kale change into particularly effective and very healthy sulforaphanes when the plants are cut. This process is a defense strategy against insects, when they hurt/bite the plant skin. The plant releases enzymes that activate the precursor substances of sulforaphanes, which are detrimental to small insects but healthy to humans. By cutting broccoli and leaving it for about thirty minutes before cooking, the natural process can be imitated.[19]

Enzymes in the intestine ensure the unlocking of component parts of food. Some plant-based ingredients can intensify or block the effects of these enzymes. That's why the effect of some medications can be increased by drinking grapefruit juice, and reduced by St. John's wort, which is also effective in treating depression.[20, 21] These enzymatic proteins, called CYP, can also play a particularly vital role during cancer treatment when the patients consume vitamin or herbal cocktails without consulting a doctor first. This can slow down the chemotherapy or make it too strong.[22]

Plants always contain a variety of substances that keep one another in check, bolstering or stopping their individual effects. This is one of the reasons why plant-based preparations generally take longer to unfold their full effect. Modern medications are based on a single active agent: That's why an aspirin pill containing 500 milligrams of acetylsalicylic acid relieves pain quite quickly while extracts of willow bark, which contain the ingredient of aspirin in addition to other substances in their natural form, need more time. But on the other hand, plant-based preparations are better tolerated and have fewer side effects.

Paradoxically, in Europe herbal medicine has been punished for this multi-target principle and better tolerance. In the 1980s, numerous preparations disappeared from the market because as a mixture of active agents they were unable to provide the required proof of an individual active agent. In 2004, European legislation made it a little easier to obtain approval, but herbal medications were withheld from cost reimbursement by large health insurance companies. The justification was that due to their very good tolerability they don't have to be classified as available only on prescription. That's why patients in Europe today have to pay for a very tolerable plant-based drug out of their own pockets while the chemical version that carries more side effects is usually covered by insurance.

Many people are interested in herbal plant-based medicines and willing to bear the costs themselves. But still, the right dosage and high-quality preparations are important here. Please do consult with your physician or pharmacist. Details are important when aiming for optimum herbal medicine treatment. During my consultation hours, I often hear about failed attempts of trying to find sleep with the aid of valerian extracts, for example. When I inquire about this further, it often turns out that the dose taken was far under the necessary dose of 600 milligrams for valerian—in which case valerian simply can't work.

The severe side effects that conventional single-ingredient drugs (such as cortisone, antirheumatics, or pain medication) often cause are rarely questioned, whereas people are particularly critical when it comes to the side effects of medicinal plants. This can be seen in the case of kava kava, which is an effective help against anxiety and nervousness and which was withdrawn from sale in 2002 due to reputed severe liver damage in some patients, then approved again, then banned once more. Now it's been approved yet again. The liver damage, as it turned out, was most likely not tied to the drug at all.

St. John's wort is fighting a similar battle. Many studies have proven that St. John's wort is an effective treatment option for slight to medium depression. Moreover, it has fewer side effects than chemical antidepressants. Since it activates the CYP-enzyme path in the liver, St. John's wort can, however, enhance the breakdown of other medications taken at the same time. That's why it shouldn't be used when certain other drugs have been prescribed.[23] But many patients are so unsure after reading the numerous press reports that they assume St. John's wort is dangerous in general. That's definitely not the case. (And we mustn't forget that other preparations, too, have their respective interactions.) St. John's wort is an excellent plant-based medication for the treatment of depression when the possibility of drug interaction is taken into account.

## EFFECTIVE THERAPIES USING MEDICINAL PLANTS

The versatility of medicinal plants can be seen in another therapeutic area in which St. John's wort can be used. Applied to the skin, the oily extract of St. John's wort, the "red oil" (named because of its red color), has a topical anti-inflammatory effect.[24] You can try using it for skin inflammations or bruises.

In Ayurveda and in Traditional Chinese Medicine, numerous plants and their extracts are combined and used, even in severe, complex diseases. In Germany, it's predominantly individual plant extracts that are used—analogously to the synthetic medications—for the targeted treatment of symptoms or health problems mainly in less severe illnesses. Thereby only a fraction of the potential effect of herbal medicine can be achieved.

The domain of medicinal plant therapy in Germany are coughs and sneezes:

- Extracts of ivy, primrose, buckhorn, or thyme help against coughs.
- Sage, thyme, cress, and horseradish help against sore throats.
- Cranberries prevent, and bearberry leaves help against, inflammations of the bladder.

In 2016, two studies were published on the use of cranberry extracts to counteract inflammations of the bladder, with confusingly contradictory results, causing a lot of media discussion. One large-scale study showed that middle-aged women with chronic inflammations of the bladder actually did suffer fewer infections when they drank cranberry juice regularly.[25] In a smaller study published only a few weeks later, it turned out that cranberry extract was ineffective in treating an already existing, severe, purulent inflammation of the bladder in patients in a nursing home over the age of eighty-five.[26] Many media sources then issued a blanket claim that cranberry was generally ineffective to treat inflammations of the bladder. The small, but crucial difference remained unmentioned: Cranberry helps to prevent—but not to treat.

Orthopedic and organic diseases can be treated with the right medicinal plants:

- Special tree bark extracts or rampion help in arthroses and back pain.
- Psyllium husk helps against inflammations of the bowel.

- Stomachaches from irritable bowel syndrome can be alleviated with myrrh and peppermint oil.

Peppermint oil generally relaxes the muscles in the gastro-intestinal tract and can thus prevent painful cramps. That's why it's recommended to take peppermint oil capsules or drops before a colonoscopy. However, the muscle-relaxing effect can cause heartburn as a side effect since the esophageal sphincter that sits between the stomach and the esophagus is loosened.

Medicinal plants are also useful for:

- migraine prevention (butterbur and wild chamomile)
- gynecological hormonal discomforts (black snakeroot and monk's pepper)
- heart diseases (hawthorn)
- liver disorders (milk thistle)

Of the countless plants and plant compounds that are used in China and India, only a few have made it to the European market in the form of medications so far. Ginseng, for example, is used as a nutritional supplement in the complementary treatment of diabetes mellitus. The plant-based medicinal product PADMA 28, which contains more than twenty plant-based individual substances and is from Tibetan medicine, is now produced as a drug in Switzerland and has become well known. A few smaller studies were able to prove the effectiveness of PADMA 28 in diseases that occur due to calcification of leg arteries,[27] and many patients to whom I've recommended PADMA 28 have experienced an alleviation of their symptoms. Yet still, this plant-based medication has not been able to assert itself among specialist physicians.

It's difficult for plants that, despite having a long tradition, haven't been researched in a sufficient number of studies. For the treatment of rheumatism with incense there is only limited data available, and due to a lack of funding this is not going to be rectified in the foreseeable future. And so, I only recommend incense as a second choice in case conventional medicine doesn't achieve a sufficiently positive effect or can't be tolerated. One patient suffered from pain in the joints and swelling day in and day out, despite taking different antirheumatics. Then she took, following the recommendation from her rheumatologist, six capsules of incense every day—and her symptoms improved immensely. Naturally, an individual case like this is not scientific proof, but it does emphasize the need to pay attention to the potential of phytotherapy.

For me, phytotherapy plays a significant role in medicine. The body knows plants. In the early stages of illness in patients who are sensitive to chemical pharmaceuticals, a therapy with medicinal plants can support healing without interfering too much with the body's regulation. This takes time. That said, if the medications show no effect after three months, I advise my patients to discontinue them.

Studies from China and India show the extent of the potential there is to tap. Chinese medicinal plant therapy is effective in treating dementia, irritable bowel syndrome, rheumatism, or vascular diseases.[28] But it may take another few years before Chinese and Ayurvedic medicinal plant therapy can be evaluated better and more safely.

## The Fifteen Most Important Areas of Application of Phytomedicine

- Anxiety disorders and stress: lavender
- Depression: amber
- Sleep disorders: valerian, lemon balm, passion flower, hops

- Liver diseases: milk thistle
- Cardiac insufficiency: hawthorn
- Diabetes: ginseng
- Atherosclerosis, intermittent claudication: PADMA 28
- Inflammations of the bladder: nasturtium, horseradish, cranberries, bearberry leaves
- Irritable colon: peppermint oil, fennel, caraway, anise
- Inflammation of the bowel: myrrh, psyllium husk, tormentil
- Migraine: wild chamomile, butterbur (migraine prevention)
- Tension headache: mint oil (applied locally)
- Arthrosis: rosehip extracts, tree bark extracts (e.g., willow bark), turmeric
- Early-stage dementia: saffron, ginkgo
- Cancer (supplementary therapy): mistletoe

# CHAPTER NINE

# My Treatment Methods

*Treating Eight Common Chronic Diseases Successfully*

Severe chronic diseases aren't easy to treat. They often require the continuous intake of heavy medications or invasive surgical procedures, which can be significantly helpful but also carry a lot of side effects. As part of integrative medicine, which combines naturopathy with conventional medicine, we strive to treat our patients with as few side effects as possible and to use lifestyle changes to optimize their convalescence and hopefully even reach a full recovery, "de-chronification." It is then often possible to lower the dose of medications. But this requires a certain self-discipline and awareness. Patience is also necessary, because what has been building up for a long time in symptoms and illness needs time to disappear. Especially so if one wishes to avoid severe side effects.

The following pages illustrate the different paths conventional medicine and naturopathy take, where they harmonize well with one another, and where they take different approaches, using eight common chronic diseases as examples. The list of my "Top Ten" for each disease makes no claims of being complete and is not ordered according to any priorities. It is not a substitute for a conversation with your physician.

## HYPERTENSION

Hypertension has become a widespread disease in Western societies. Roughly 40 percent of adults and more than 80 percent of those over the age of sixty-five are suffering from it.[1] Studies among indigenous peoples show that hypertension practically doesn't exist in those communities initially, but becomes frequent with the introduction of a Western lifestyle.[2, 3] This is a clear indication that hypertension is predominantly the consequence of a certain lifestyle. Obesity, consumption of alcohol, lack of exercise, stress, and a bad diet that contains too much animal protein, animal fats, salt, and too few vegetables and fruit are all factors that cause hypertension. Usually these factors add up so that hypertension is less a disease but rather a symptom of the overexertion of the body.

### Treatment Approach of Conventional Medicine

There are several very good medications with which hypertension can be treated effectively. But for quite a few patients these medications don't work (the patients are "resistant to therapy"), while others suffer from side effects. Modern and elaborate treatment methods, on the other hand, interfere in the body. For instance, the nerves of the renal arteries can be atrophied with a catheter (hormones and secretion performance of the kidneys play a role in hypertension). Another road of treatment is the implantation of pacemakers at the carotid arteries. Both procedures, however, have not yet delivered any scientific proof for their effectiveness. It seems a little absurd to me to treat a disease that is predominantly dependent on lifestyle with invasive technological and costly methods—especially if they are not accompanied by a change in lifestyle.

## Treatment Approach of Naturopathic Medicine

There are plenty of naturopathic approaches to therapy whose effectiveness is scientifically substantiated and that work in practice. Of course, an individualized approach must be taken: Some people have high blood pressure even though they exercise, due to their genes and meat-based diet. In that case, more exercise is futile, and only a change in diet can help. Medication may still be necessary. Other people have an excellent diet but suffer from continuous stress in their job—in that case the biggest successes are achieved with meditation, tai chi, and yoga. Some foods not only lower blood pressure, but are also healthy for the heart. Walnuts, for example, protect the vessels, and flaxseed and psyllium lower the LDL cholesterol level, which is a risk factor for a heart attack or a stroke. Since inflammations in the mouth, as well as parodontitis, carry a heightened risk for subsequent vascular diseases (the bacteria travel through the body), I always ask patients about the condition of their teeth and recommend dental hygiene, a thorough cleaning technique, and regular flossing.

## My Top Ten for Hypertension

- A vegetarian or vegan diet: Substitute meat with vegetables, tofu, and soy, as soy protein lowers blood pressure. If you don't want to give up cheese and milk, you should at least severely limit the amount you consume.

- Therapeutic fasting: It's effective to practice therapeutic fasting twice a year and/or fast intermittently, e.g., fourteen hours of prolonged night-fasting.
- Superfoods: Among them are vegetables containing nitrate, such as beetroot (if you want to consume it in the form of juice, you should drink at least 8.5 ounces a day), spinach, and arugula; walnuts and pistachios (unsalted); as well as flaxseed. Use either shredded flaxseed or grind it up yourself. Flaxseed oil can also lower the blood pressure, but if you eat whole flaxseeds, you will profit from its additional health-promoting effects (such as prevention of breast and prostate cancer). Blueberries, which you can eat fresh, frozen, or as a powder, also lower elevated blood pressure. Ideally, you should eat one of these food products once a day.
- Superdrinks: Drink two to three cups of hibiscus or green tea every day. After having hibiscus tea, you should drink some water or rinse your mouth since the acid it contains can damage the dental enamel.
- Native, fruity olive oil: Use it in large quantities if possible. Extracts from olive leaves also lower the blood pressure, but they have to be taken in the form of pills—chewing the leaves is not enough.
- Meditation: I recommend meditating for at least thirty minutes every day.
- Yoga and tai chi/qigong: Practice in a class once a week and every second day for fifteen minutes at home.
- Bloodletting or donating blood: Either one is effective for people with elevated ferritin levels or "thick blood" (elevated hematocrit, which your GP can measure by doing blood work).
- Exercise and/or endurance sports: Ideally, you should exercise for 150 to 300 minutes every week.
- Regular hydrotherapy: Most effective here are Scotch hose treatments (note that after a heart attack, a resting period of three weeks is

necessary) and temperature-increasing arm and sauna baths (without using the cold immersion bath), once a day if possible.

## CORONARY HEART DISEASE AND ARTERIOSCLEROSIS

Cardiovascular diseases are among the most common diseases in humans. For many years, they have been one of the leading causes of death in the industrialized world. Coronary heart disease develops over the course of many years before a blood clot actually obstructs a damaged part of a vessel, which then causes a heart attack or a stroke. That's why one of the cornerstones of therapy in this case is the treatment of individual risk factors such as hypertension, diabetes, or lipid metabolic disorder, particularly, heightened LDL cholesterol levels. The most important measure to take when suffering from this vascular disease is to quit smoking.

### Treatment Approach of Conventional Medicine

Over the past three decades, cardiology has undergone impressive successes. Today, a supportive stent can be placed with the aid of catheters at the afflicted coronary vessel in an acute heart attack to prevent further damage of the heart muscle. Heart valve defects can also be treated via catheters. However, these technical interventions and advancements don't influence the underlying vascular disease, the arteriosclerosis. The renowned American cardiologist Eric J. Topol called treating coronary heart disease without a heart attack with balloon dilatation and stents "medical cosmetics."[4] And it's true: If the original disease—the arteriosclerosis—isn't tackled with a change in lifestyle and with medication, the patient's life expectancy isn't prolonged by the procedure. To make matters more complicated, heart attacks don't develop at the very narrow places, but usually at early-stage stenoses where there is only a slight constriction. Many patients who undergo a heart catheter examination aren't even aware of this fact. It's possible that physicians don't convey this, but maybe it's that people, out of sheer enthusiasm for the technology, don't want to hear that the disease continues to exist. But it can also have to do with the fact that men are more likely to suffer from a heart attack than women, and cardiology and cardiac surgery are male-dominated specialties. Men tend to favor technical solutions.

## Treatment Approach of Naturopathic Medicine

Naturopathy focuses mainly on a change of lifestyle with a vegetarian, high-fiber diet and a lot of exercise. Water treatments using hot and cold water in turn are useful to train the vessels. Exercise through stamina training and conscious periods of rest, supported by targeted and very regular relaxation techniques, are important, as well as yoga, mindfulness exercises, or meditation. Since stress is a great risk factor for heart attacks, stress reduction plays a pivotal part in heart diseases. Medicinal plants like hawthorn can help with slight cardiac insufficiency.

## My Top Ten for Coronary Heart Disease and Arteriosclerosis

- Vegan diet: Even though nowadays all patients are prescribed a fat-reducing drug after a heart attack, it's quite possible (even though the opposite is often claimed) to achieve a similar effect with an extensive change in diet. Olive oil and walnuts have a particularly protective effect on the vessels. Therapeutic fasting is good, but not during the first three months after a heart attack. Sometimes the heightened LDL cholesterol levels are genetically determined, in which case diet, as healthy as it may be, can unfortunately only help very little.

- Moderate exercise therapy: It's good to have a varied exercise program with stamina training that isn't focused on high performance and that also contains other elements, especially playful forms of exercise such as tai chi.

- Yoga: According to studies, yoga not only lowers heart risk in general, it also reduces the intensity and the duration of atrial fibrillation, a frequent cardiac arrhythmia (Iyengar yoga is best in this case).[5] Breathing slowly as part of yogic practices improves the symptoms of cardiac insufficiency.

- Heart superfoods: The frequent consumption of certain foods can successfully lower LDL cholesterol levels. These foods include almonds, flaxseed, and oats, as well as walnuts, which ensure greater elasticity of the vessels. Particularly surprising is that the daily consumption of (high-fat) avocado also lowers LDL cholesterol levels since this fruit contains simple unsaturated fatty acids similar to that of olive oil. Ginger reduces other risky fats, the triglycerides.

- Plant-based omega-3 fatty acids: Flaxseed oil, flaxseed, canola oil, walnuts, green leafy vegetables, soy oil, wheat germ oil, algae, and algae extracts provide these vessel-protecting fatty acids.

- Garlic: Though it only minimally lowers the blood pressure and the cholesterol levels, garlic does improve elasticity of the vessels.

- Pomegranate juice: The juice and extracts of the pomegranate have the highest antioxidant effect of all plant-based juices. One study was able to show that the repeated consumption of pomegranate increased blood flow to the heart.[6] It also lowers blood pressure and cholesterol levels.

- Dark chocolate: It reduces the risk of vascular diseases slightly (and tastes good).

- Dental health: Dental abscesses and periodontitis are accompanied by a heightened risk of vascular diseases like heart attacks. Similar to cases of hypertension, I always ask patients with cardiovascular diseases or diabetes about the state of their dental health and recommend regular dental prophylaxis (dental cleaning).
- Sauna and Kneipp treatments: Water treatments help treat cardiac insufficiency and vascular diseases. Regular visits to the sauna can—according to a Finnish study—protect from life-threatening cardiac arrhythmias.[7] But the temperatures should not be too high (and the sauna visit not too long). Heliotherapy, meaning moderate sun bathing, is also a part of heart protection. However, sunburn should be avoided at all costs. It's better to take short sunbaths between April and September (if you live in the northern hemisphere).

## ARTHROSIS

The fact that we are now living longer contributes to us developing more arthroses. But in an arthrosis, wear and tear due to overstraining isn't the decisive issue (with some exceptions, such as high-performance athletes, for example). Even though we tend to perform work that is much less physically straining than we did only one hundred years ago, arthroses nevertheless occur more frequently. The crucial factors today are bad diet, obesity, and lack of exercise. From the age of sixty onward, half of all women and one in three men in the Western world are affected by arthrosis.[8] Arthrosis begins with an inflammation and the attrition of articular cartilage. The chronic pain, however, only occurs many years later. It is caused by a complex interplay of bad posture, muscular deterioration and shortening, irritated tendons and ligaments continuously trying to stabilize the joint, as well as dysfunctional pain processing in the brain.

## Treatment Approach of Conventional Medicine

Conventional medicine recommends a normalization of weight for obese people and employs physical therapy to achieve this. Subsequently, physical treatments are prescribed, with cold, heat, and electricity—they have a detumescent effect and relieve the symptoms. Pain medication often includes nonsteroidal anti-inflammatory drugs (NSAIDs), which can, however, lead to severe side effects. Ibuprofen and Diclofenac, for example, have come under criticism because of the potential kidney damage, heightened heart risks, and asthma they can cause. When these medications are taken over a prolonged period of time, there is great danger of kidney failure, which may even lead to the need for dialysis; gastric bleeding occurs frequently. Good physical therapy may be able to alleviate the symptoms, but usually surgery is necessary at some stage. An artificial joint replacement (endoprosthesis) is implanted, often to great effect, in arthroses of the hips. Knee endoprosthesis, on the other hand, is more complicated and not as successful as hip endoprosthesis.

## Treatment Approach of Naturopathic Medicine

Arthrosis is an important domain of traditional therapy methods from India, China, and Europe. Particularly when it comes to arthrosis of the knees, they are very effective in relieving symptoms and improving mobility and resilience. They can help delay the joint replacement procedure. But if other areas of the body are increasingly affected by the arthrosis, e.g., the back due to problems with the hips, or the shoulders due to walking with a cane, a surgical-orthopedic treatment becomes necessary.

### My Top Ten for Arthrosis

- Leech therapy: Particularly in arthrosis of the knees, but also in osteoarthritis of the thumb or arthrosis of the shoulder, this method can often alleviate symptoms, have a detumescent effect, and improve function for months at a time.
- Acupuncture: It relieves pain, but because the effect is not lasting, you should go in for acupuncture treatments on a regular basis, especially in arthroses of the knees and shoulders.
- Ayurveda: With its multimodal approach, Ayurveda is well-suited to relieve pain and improve functionality, particularly in arthroses of the knees.
- Cupping: The effect is not as pronounced as that of leech therapy or Ayurveda, but it can help temporarily.
- Physical and moderate exercise therapy: It strengthens the muscles, especially in arthroses of the knees, hips, or shoulders. It must be performed regularly under supervision and also practiced at home.
- Medicinal plants: Use rosehip extracts (only cold extracts are effective, which is why rosehip tea doesn't help, unfortunately), rampion, or tree bark extracts internally. Comfrey, wolf's bane, or amber oil are suitable for external application. Phytotherapy has a mild effect, but it can be used as a supplement.
- Therapeutic fasting: It can reduce chronic pain caused by arthrosis. Apart from the anti-inflammatory effect of fasting, the weight reduction generally shows a beneficial effect immediately. Since the transition to a healthy, plant-based diet is easier after fasting, it is a sustainable supplementary therapy method.

- Plant-based, vegetarian diet: In obese patients, this helps normalize weight. By adopting a plant-based, vegetarian diet, you avoid the intake of pro-inflammatory arachidonic acid, an unsaturated fatty acid contained in meat, fish, and eggs.
- Application of cabbage leaves or fenugreek: These common domestic remedies are effective. They are easy to do at home and according to a study, they are just as effective as ointments that contain Diclofenac.[9]
- Heat and cold therapy: Local warm applications like fango and peloid packs, hay bags, or cold quark poultices are suitable here. A systemic therapy in a cold chamber is also recommended.

## DEPRESSION AND ANXIETY SYNDROMES

Depression is on the rise in Germany as well as in the United States.[10] The causes are manifold, many questions remain unsolved. Every fourth to fifth patient visits their GP because they are suffering from a mild or moderate depression.[11]

### Treatment Approach of Conventional Medicine

The most common treatment is—apart from psychotherapy—drug-based. It's mainly tricyclic antidepressants and selective serotonin reuptake inhibitors that are being prescribed. But in the scientific review of the effectiveness of these drugs, many studies are overlooked—almost half of them. It's not hard to guess that the overlooked studies are those that were unable to show that treatment with antidepressants was more effective compared to treatment with a placebo. Overall, then, the impact of these antidepressants is based largely on the placebo effect. Peter Gøtzsche, director of the Nordic Cochrane Center in Copenhagen, questions the effectiveness of antidepressants entirely.[12] I wouldn't go that far. In severe depression, it's a blessing to have these medications available. In the much more common milder depressions, however, I think preference should be given to naturopathic and integrative methods, because many antidepressants lead to weight gain and numerous subsequent problems. Other antidepressants have come under criticism, since they possibly increase suicide rate and cause addictions.[13] So, it is high time for more naturopathy to be used in the treatment of depressions.

## Treatment Approach of Naturopathic Medicine

Depression has many causes: it can be biographical, situational, biochemical, or due to lifestyle. From a naturopathic point of view, depression is caused by many factors and not just by a malfunction of receptors and neurotransmitters, to which biological psychiatry tries to narrow it down. Naturopathy can address many of these levels simultaneously. If, for example, one doesn't consider body and soul to be separate entities, it is obvious that a healthy diet and sufficient exercise as well as stress-reducing practices affect a person's mood. Medicinal plants such as amber can have a mood-enhancing effect. Acupuncture helps against anxiety. Mind-body medicine provides exercises through which, if they are carried out regularly, the balance of neurotransmitters in the brain is changed in a positive way. Similarly, light, touch, and spirituality are possible starting points.

## My Top Ten for Depression and Anxiety Syndromes

- Exercise and physical activity: Even though it takes a lot of effort to exercise or engage in physical activity when you are suffering from depression, it is worth it—serotonin levels increase and the processing of noradrenalin in the brain is improved. In addition, exercise facilitates the growth of new nerve cells. It's not that important what you do, but that you do it regularly.

- Experiencing nature, "forest bathing," and gardening: When it is done in nature, every form of exercise seems to help counteract depression even better.

- Yoga: Most studies confirm—no matter which disease they are concerned with—that yoga has a distinct mood-enhancing effect. Even with depression, we find a clear therapeutic effect. It's important to find a yoga technique that you like and that doesn't demand too much of you.

- Light and sun therapy: White-light therapy is particularly effective in seasonal depression, meaning depressive disorders that occur more frequently over the dark winter months. There are special lamps for this that achieve a luminosity of 10,000 lux over a distance of ten to twenty inches, so that you don't have to look directly into the light but can eat, talk on the phone, or have breakfast while bathing in the light. Thirty minutes a day are recommended, with a spectrum that resembles sunlight. The effect is greatest when the treatment is carried out between half past seven and half past eight in the morning and sets in after about a week. People who know about their propensity for winter depressions should ideally start the therapy as early as October. Sunbaths (not too frequent and without getting sunburnt) are also mood-enhancing. Sun beds can support antidepressant treatment.

- Kneipp therapy: The various water treatments stimulate the autonomic nervous system and thus foster motivation and improve the mood. Alternating Scotch hose treatments, compresses, and full-body baths can be combined with calming (lavender, melissa) or stimulating (rosemary, ginger) plant extracts.

- Heat therapy and therapeutic hyperthermia: One single systemic hyperthermic treatment with a special machine lifts the mood for about two weeks. If this is not a possibility for you, you should visit a sauna regularly. (Coldness also has a similar effect. There is no satisfying scientific data on this available yet, but the experiences in rheumatology centers with cold chambers indicate an antidepressant effect.)

- Medicinal plants: Amber is effective in mild to moderate depressions. It's important here to be aware of its interaction with other drugs—talk to your doctor about this. In Ayurvedic medicine, ashwagandha (winter cherry or poison gooseberry) has an anxiolytic and mood-enhancing effect, and in European naturopathy the same is achieved by using lavender extracts. Extracts of ginseng or roseroot can help with exhaustion. By the way, in mild depression, aromatherapy is helpful, too—lavender, rosemary, or saffron are suitable essences for an aroma lamp or for an aroma bath.

- Meditation and mindfulness training: Mild depression, burn-out, or other chronic fatigue syndromes are the result of prolonged stress. Mindfulness training or mantra meditations can help restore strength and show ways of handling the stress of life differently.

- Massages: Different massage techniques show good symptomatic effects in depression and anxiety syndromes. Subcutaneous reflex therapy, rhythmic massage (which has its origins in Anthroposophy), and Ayurvedic massages are particularly effective. This is presumably also due to the mere touch that is part of these methods, which is healing in many respects. But Ayurveda seems to be helpful in the treatment of depressions in other ways, too.

- Therapeutic fasting and diet: Therapeutic fasting can show an astonishing effect in mild depressions. Where severe depressions are concerned, one should be cautious, however, and only fast in exceptional cases in a clinic that has experience with it. Presently, nutritional therapy is being discovered as a potentially important therapeutic approach by psychiatry: For some time now, studies have been showing that an unhealthy diet with too much animal fat, sugar, and little fruit and vegetables goes hand in hand with an increasing number of depressions.[14] By now, it has also become apparent that the transition to a plant-based and wholesome diet actually does lead to an improvement of a person's mood and the reduction of depressive moods quite quickly. Not all of the details are clarified yet, but it seems, for example, that lycopene (a phytochemical) contained in tomatoes, leafy greens, and legumes as well as lentils and beans plays a major role in this.[15] Some foods, such as cocoa, bananas, cashews, and dates, provide the substance from which the happiness hormone serotonin is created. Avoiding meat, eggs, and fish reduces the intake of arachidonic acid, which leads to more depressive moods—probably because of its pro-inflammatory effect. The brain doesn't translate slight inflammatory impulses to pain, but to depression.

Those who don't want to become vegetarians or vegans should turn to a Mediterranean diet, which consists of large amounts of vegetables, fruit, and healthy fats. Omega-3 fatty acids have antidepressant effects—they are found in flaxseed oil and flaxseed, canola oil, soy, and walnuts. By the way, some studies show that artificial sweeteners are connected to increasing depressiveness.[16] So please don't try to reduce your sugar intake by switching to Diet Coke, for example.

### BACK AND NECK PAIN

Up to 85 percent of Germans suffer from persistent back pain at least once in their life, and 34 percent of Germans complain about recurrent or chronic back pain. The numbers in the United States are not far off.[17] In the Western world in general, millions of people visit a doctor every year because of back pain. In about 80 percent of the patients, the prescribed methods work initially, but very frequently the pain returns.[18, 19]

## Treatment Approach of Conventional Medicine

For a long time now, the great number of back surgeries carried out in Germany has been criticized. For many years, the cause of chronic back pain was attributed to signs of wear and tear in the bones or disc protrusions, until studies were able to demonstrate that these medical findings, which almost every person shows after a certain age, are often not even the cause of the pain.[20] That's why a surgery is unable to produce relief in many cases. It's only necessary in cases of a severe spinal disk herniation that disrupts bladder or bowel function or causes paralysis, and in cases of severe spinal stenosis (constriction of the vertebral canal), which causes great pain and can't be improved through naturopathic treatments or physical therapy. Most patients receive medication or injections with pain-killing or muscle-relaxing agents; even antidepressants are prescribed. All of these medications have, when taken for a prolonged period of time, significant side effects.

## Treatment Approach of Naturopathic Medicine

Most people suffer from "unspecific" back pain, for which naturopathic methods are highly recommended and scientifically funded. By now, the realization has prevailed that back pain shouldn't immediately be treated with injections and medication, but rather with active measures that can be carried out by the patients themselves. Since pain causes a fear of movement (kinesophobia), the gentle and conscious movement methods of yoga or tai chi are particularly suitable.

Many surgeries would become superfluous if naturopathic methods were applied consistently.

## My Top Ten for Back and Neck Pain

- Yoga: The exercises are very healing for back pain, and usually they are also better than any other therapies. Iyengar yoga and Vini yoga are particularly recommendable.
- Physical therapy and physical activity: There are specially developed back training programs that combine muscle building and stretching. Get advice on this from your orthopedist. A good manual therapy, without the "cracking" and only using gentle techniques, can also be an effective supplementary treatment. Methods like the Alexander technique put special emphasis on conscious sequences of movements in the spine. Curative eurythmy from anthroposophical medicine combines movement and breathing with talking. In a forthcoming study conducted by our work group, eurythmy proved equal to intensive physical therapy and yoga.
- Acupuncture and bed of nails: The effectiveness of acupuncture in treating back pain has been proven.[21] It can provide a good bridge until an exercise program begins; additionally, it makes it possible to perform the exercises with less pain. At home, you can use the "bed of nails," also called a "fakir mat" or an acupressure mat—a mat with small, pointy attachments that lowers the body's sensitivity to pain. It's easy to use: first, press your hands into it, then place it under the part of the back that causes pain, and remain lying on it for as long as it feels good.
- Leech therapy: A recently concluded study by my group demonstrated the beneficial effect of a single treatment with leeches. In comparison to physical therapy, the pain receded significantly more after eight weeks.[22] The long-term effect has not been sufficiently

researched, but in otherwise treatment-resistant pain, I definitely recommend at least trying it.

- Walking barefoot: Back pain is not only an issue of the back. The entire "motion apparatus" is interconnected. That's why foot or knee problems can also cause back pain. Experienced physical therapists, manual therapists, and osteopaths know these connections. It's recommendable to mobilize the fasciae from the sole of the foot using, for example, a spiky massage ball (but step on it forcefully, since it has to hurt a little . . .)

- Standing: Avoid sitting for hours on end. Take walks whenever you can, and work at a standing desk or a vertically adjustable table.

- Meditation: When stress is one of the causes of back pain—and it often is—mindfulness and mantra meditations (such as Jyoti) often help.

- Heat therapy: Tense muscles can be loosened by using warmth, even at home. The simplest method is to take a hot bath. You can also buy heat packs at the pharmacy or online, e.g., peloid packs, beeswax packs, grain and ginger sacks. An alternative to a hot water bottle are heat plasters or capsaicin (Spanish pepper)—however, both irritate the skin and aren't tolerated by everybody.

- Cupping: In all its forms (wet, dry, or as a massage), cupping usually helps to treat back pain quite effectively. For household use, dry cupping and the cupping massage can be carried out by your partner.

- Diet: Therapeutic fasting helps us lose superfluous weight, and to transition to a vegetarian diet. A base-rich diet (vegetables, fruit, sprouts) is advisable, since meat, fish, dairy products, and grains contain acid and can have a negative impact on the connective tissue. Eat less bread and drink mineral water that is rich in bicarbonate.

## DIABETES

Diabetes is causing more and more concern for physicians and health officials. For years, the number of cases has been on the rise in Europe and the United States.[23] While it was mainly the elderly who were affected before ("adult-onset diabetes"), type 2 diabetes patients are becoming younger year by year.[24] Almost all scientists agree that malnutrition, overeating, and obesity are responsible for the epidemic, combined with a lack of physical activity (things are different for type 1 diabetes, where the insulin-producing cells are destroyed by the immune system). All attempts of prevention have been futile. According to recent reports, diabetes affects 9.4 percent of the population of the United States, or about 30.3 million people. Approximately 90 percent of all diabetes cases are type 2 diabetes. In addition, another 34 percent of American adults—84 million people—have prediabetes.[25]

### Treatment Approach of Conventional Medicine

There are drugs that not only lower elevated blood sugar levels, but also significantly reduce the actual danger for diabetes patients (such as dying from heart attack, stroke, or kidney disease). Metformin is the drug used most frequently; it facilitates cells' glucose absorption and thus lowers blood sugar levels. The next step is insulin therapy, which leads to weight gain, however, and often causes a vicious cycle: The patients move less, which further disrupts the metabolism and carries new health risks with it. New drugs like Empagliflozin and Liraglutide pursue different modes of action, such as the increased secretion of glucose via the urine. Further medications are in the pipeline. But as is so often the case, highly effective new drugs have two disadvantages: They cause side effects and they are expensive.

## Treatment Approach of Naturopathic Medicine

Intensive lifestyle therapies and fasting try to normalize the insulin balance, to stabilize it, and to minimize the risk factors that are the result of the illness. A change in diet and exercise are important pillars. Bloodletting can be useful as a supplementary treatment.

## My Top Ten for Diabetes

- Oat days: Oatmeal lowers blood sugar levels. Eating nothing but oatmeal on certain days is a moderate form of fasting and brings relief to the metabolism.
- Vegan diet: Studies show that the beneficial effect of a vegan diet is demonstrated clearly for diabetes mellitus.[26]
- Nuts and olive oil: They should be consumed every day. They lower the risk of cardiovascular diseases by protecting the vessels.
- Intermittent fasting and therapeutic fasting: One study was able to show that 16/8 fasting—i.e., a daily sixteen-hour abstention from food—improves blood values and even fatty livers within a few weeks.[27] Prolonged therapeutic fasting of seven to ten days (twice a year) has even stronger effects.[28] It's best to combine both.
- Bloodletting: It lowers blood pressure, intensifies insulin's effect, and normalizes sugar metabolism by lowering ferritin levels. It's particularly suited for patients with a fatty liver, which often develops in patients with diabetes.
- Ayurveda: In India, multimodal therapy concepts (adjusted to the individual patient) are employed to remarkable success.
- Ginseng: Traditional Chinese Medicine attributes a vital energy-maintaining power to this legendary medicinal plant. Its effects have best been proven in the treatment of diabetes mellitus. That's why trying it can be recommended as a supplementary measure.

- Vinegar: Consuming vinegar with a meal (i.e., in pickled vegetables or taken with a spoon) lowers the rise of blood sugar levels after eating.
- Legumes: A daily ration of chickpeas, lentils, or beans leads to improved blood sugar regulation.
- Avoid fattening chemicals (obesogens): Environmental toxins, such as the so-called persistent organic pollutants (POPs), are stored in the fat tissue. At the same time, they seem to cause weight gain, even though this has not yet been proven conclusively. Since they build up continuously along the food chain, they are contained to 90 percent in animal products, first and foremost in salmon and tuna.[29] They are best avoided by switching to a vegan diet.

## RHEUMATISM

Rheumatoid arthritis, formerly called polyarthritis, is accompanied by painful inflammations and swelling of the joints. It leads to severe damage of the joints if treated insufficiently.

### Treatment Approach of Conventional Medicine

Up until a few decades ago, doctors were relatively powerless in the face of rheumatoid arthritis. Now, many new, effective drugs are available, the most famous among them is Methotrexate. Almost every year new biologicals (substances developed with the aid of biotechnology) come on the market, and they usually achieve a significant improvement, especially in combination with Methotrexate. Still, these medications don't cure the disease. A lot of the time, cortisone has to be taken also—accompanied by the well-known side effects such as weight gain, increased blood pressure, a rise in blood sugar levels, etc.

## Treatment Approach of Naturopathic Medicine

The treatment of rheumatism is a good example of an integrative medicine in which effective conventional medicine is combined with naturopathy. We cannot forgo modern antirheumatics and biologicals, since the effects of naturopathic methods are ultimately not strong enough. But they are appropriate supplements: They relieve symptoms and can facilitate a reduction of the dosage of medications. It's important to start using them at the very beginning of the illness without delay. In my experience, stress plays a negative role in rheumatoid arthritis as well as in other autoimmune diseases.

## My Top Ten for Rheumatism

- Fasting: Numerous studies demonstrate the symptom-relieving effect of fasting.[30] Every day at the Immanuel Hospital, the biggest rheumatology center in Berlin, we see good results from fasting.
- Mediterranean and plant-based diet: It's important to prolong the effect of fasting by adopting an anti-inflammatory diet for as long as possible afterward. Patients should refrain from eating meat and eggs completely, since they contain pro-inflammatory arachidonic acid. Dairy products should be consumed only in small quantities. Whether a strictly vegan diet provides further advantages is not scientifically resolved.
- Elimination diet: Many patients have found that certain foods can cause a rheumatic episode. Often, these are meats or dairy products, but not exclusively. If a worsening of the condition has been noted multiple times after consuming certain foods, they should be avoided. However, this is subject to change, which is why it's possible to test the suspected foods again after a while.

- Mindfulness meditation: In three studies, regular mindfulness meditation led to a better mental state in patients with rheumatism. In one of the studies, inflammatory activity was also diminished. Meditation as a method of reducing stress is especially recommendable if the beginning of the disease was connected to an exhausting life phase or a difficult event.[31]

- Cryotherapy: Cold chambers, localized ice packs, or cooling quark poultices relieve joint pain very well.

- Medicinal herbs: Initial studies have shown that turmeric has an anti-inflammatory effect.[32] I recommend turmeric in its natural form (put two teaspoons of it in your meal or a drink every day together with a pinch of black pepper, which improves absorption in the body). Extracts of stinging nettle, rampion, or incense have not been sufficiently examined by science to allow for them to be recommended as standard. If, however, there exists a resistance to therapy or if all other usual and newer antirheumatic drugs and biologicals cause particularly severe side effects, it's advisable to give them a try. Particularly with incense, we keep seeing surprising successes over and over in our hospital.

- Omega-3 fatty acids: They have an anti-inflammatory effect which can be used as a supplementary treatment in rheumatism. Plant-based sources that contain alpha-linolenic acid (flaxseed, flaxseed oil, canola oil, soy oil, walnuts, leafy greens, etc.), are recommendable. In principle, fatty saltwater fish are also a good source of omega-3 fatty acids, in this case for the long-chain fatty acids EPA (eicosapentaenoic acid) and DHA (docosahexaenoic acid). But since rheumatism is often accompanied by osteoporosis, and fish can foster osteoporosis because of its acidity and is often polluted with heavy metals, I recommend plant-based sources of omega-3 fatty acids.

- Gamma-linolenic acid: It is found in borage seed, black caraway, or evening primrose oil and has an anti-inflammatory effect. Some smaller studies confirm this, but the effect is mild.[33]
- Acupuncture: For rheumatism, this healing method is recommended as pain therapy.
- Ayurveda: In India, rheumatism is often treated with Ayurvedic herbs. In an initial study, the Ayurvedic therapy was not inferior to Methotrexate.[34] This is not enough to issue a general recommendation, but an attempt can be made if other therapies are unsatisfying.

## GASTROINTESTINAL DISEASES

The digestive tract is, due to its nerve nets that span from the mouth to the anus, a sensitive area with many complex functions that react to both psychosomatic processes as well as serious metabolic disorders and infections. Common and not easily treatable diseases include esophagitis (reflux disease whose symptoms include acid reflux) and irritable bowel syndrome, which causes stomachaches and digestive problems with diarrhea, bloating, and indigestion without any abnormalities showing up during a colonoscopy.

### Treatment Approach of Conventional Medicine

Antacids—proton pump inhibitors (PPIs)—and the antibiotic treatment of the stomach bacterium *Helicobacter* have been used in the therapy of gastric ulcers and severe esophagitis with great success. However, PPIs are among the medications prescribed too often nowadays. Around the world, they are recommended by physicians generously and for excessive lengths of time, probably in more than one in every two cases without proper indication being detected.[35] This is not a trivial problem, since studies have shown that the prolonged intake of PPIs is linked to a series of serious risk increases, beginning with dementia, to cardiovascular diseases and osteoporosis.[36, 37] It's not rare that they also cause vitamin B12 deficiency, which, in turn, can result in nerve damage. Moreover, they impair the feeling of satiety while eating and can cause stomach pains, nausea, and diarrhea. Finally, the acid suppression can lead to undesirable bacteria settling in the gastrointestinal tract. Consequently, this can lead to unfavorable changes in the intestinal microbiome. That's why PPIs shouldn't be taken any longer than is necessary. A study was able to show that the body starts defending itself against the PPIs after only eight weeks: It reacts to the blocking of acids with an overproduction of the hormones facilitating acid production.[38] In 40 percent of cases, the discontinuation of the drugs is accompanied by withdrawal symptoms.[39] Previously nonexistent gastrointestinal problems develop. Thus, we see that PPIs can also be addictive.

Patients I see in consultations often report that they had been diagnosed with a diaphragmatic hernia—this is the medical term for a malfunctioning closing of the sphincter at the lower end of the esophagus where it meets the stomach. There are many people with this diagnosis, but it doesn't necessarily mean that this results in a reflux disease, meaning the rise of the gastric juices. Therefore, you shouldn't feel like you are suffering from an uncurable disease straight away. Contributing factors to the development of this hernia are obesity, stress, and lack of exercise and thus, there is the possibility for it to regress.

About 17 percent of the United States's population suffers from irritable bowel syndrome.[40] The exact cause for this is undetermined. But stress and excessive strain play a role in this, along with, probably, intestinal bacteria that contribute to a lowering of the pain threshold and to digestive problems when they settle incorrectly and even to natural intestinal movements causing problems. So far, there are no good, effective therapies that conventional medicine can offer, except for a FODMAP diet (Fermentable Oligo-, Di-, Mono-saccharides and Polyols), which avoids anything that causes flatulence and that is hard to digest.

## Treatment Approach of Naturopathic Medicine

It's useful to integrate naturopathy into the treatment of gastrointestinal diseases. The domain here is phytomedicine, but the methods of mind-body medicine, probiotics, and, of course, diet are certainly important components of the therapy. Apart from specific inflammatory bowel diseases like ulcerative colitis and Crohn's disease, it's in cases of irritable bowel disease and moderate cases of gastritis and esophagitis where a naturopathic treatment is suitable.

## My Top Ten for Gastrointestinal Diseases

*Irritable Bowel Syndrome:*

- Phytotherapy: To treat pain and spasms, peppermint oil in the form of capsules, melissa tea, or artichoke extract are helpful. Drops with fennel, caraway (also used as a wrap or ointment), as well as anise relieve flatulence. Myrrh is effective in treating diarrhea; for indigestion it's best to use psyllium seed husks and mineral waters containing sulfate. Turmeric helps in all these afflictions.
- Probiotics: Various preparations have shown effectiveness in treating irritable bowel syndrome in initial studies.[41] I recommend the already tested "classics": *lactobacilli, bifidobacterial, Escherichia coli Nissle, Enterococcus faecalis,* or bread drink.
- Mind-body medicine: In studies, relaxation techniques including meditation, yoga, hypnosis, breathing exercises, and autogenic

training have proven to be effective in treating irritable bowel syndrome.[42, 43]

- Diet: In our Ayurvedic outpatient clinic, we are constantly astonished by the positive reactions that occur when patients transform their diets according to Ayurvedic principles. Whole-food nutrition can be effective, but you should test whether you can tolerate raw foods. Beyond that, the FODMAP diet has shown successes. Here, various food groups are avoided, particularly cabbage, legumes, fruit containing large quantities of fructose, artificial sweeteners, and a few food additives, along with alcohol, wheat, and many dairy products. As an alternative I advise patients with irritable bowel syndrome to start by reducing fructose, then temporarily avoid wheat or gluten. If you feel a significant improvement after two weeks without gluten, and you suffer from less flatulence and pain, it's likely that you are intolerant to gluten or wheat, respectively, and should continue to avoid them. After a few weeks, gluten can be put to the test once more, because some people experience a temporary sensitivity caused by stress, the aftermath of an infection, alcohol, or antibiotics. Where fructose is concerned, the hypersensitivity depends mainly on the quantity. If it's more than 50 grams a day, most people experience digestive problems. And it doesn't take long to reach that amount with a diet containing a lot of ready-made products and "naturally" sweetened foods. For diarrhea, I recommend medicinal clay, drinkable peloid, coffee charcoal, blueberries and blueberry juice, and tea with berry leaves.
- Acupuncture: It can have a good symptom-relieving effect in all forms of irritable bowel syndrome.
- Heat: It's not quite clear how hyperthermia works, but the heat seems to calm the autonomic nerves in the gastrointestinal tract. We successfully treat patients suffering from irritable bowel syndrome with it.

## Heartburn and Reflux Disease

- Bitter compounds (bitters): Extracts of bitter candytuft or chamomile boost "propulsion," i.e., the transportation of food from the stomach. Furthermore, they facilitate digestion by stimulating the bile. In addition, medicinal herbs that protect the mucosa are added to some multi-compound preparations.
- Flaxseed gruel: It calms the irritated mucosa.
- Medicinal clay: It buffers acid in the stomach.
- Avoid peppermint tea, coffee, and alcohol: They stimulate the reflux. Eat dinner early and lie down with your upper body propped up when you go to bed.

# CHAPTER TEN

# Strategies for a Healthy Life

*How to Find Your Own Way*

I f you have come this far in this book, you might find yourself wanting to change something in your life now. But you're probably asking yourself: How? Where to begin? I can't provide you with a fixed formula, because it all depends on what kind of a person you are, which symptoms you might have, what your life looks like, and what you want to achieve. But I think that you'll find plenty of information and suggestions in this book from which you can choose. Try to look at this potential of possible actions in a positive way in order to improve your quality of life and become healthier, and not as something stressful.

The basics are clear: a plant-based diet with as few animal proteins (milk, meat, fish, eggs) as possible, sufficient physical activity, ideally outside and in nature, as well as active relaxation, ideally through meditation. "Active" in the sense that most people think they are relaxing when they are simply being passive—when watching television, for example—but the lab results tell a different story. Even a sleeping person doesn't relax as much as a meditating person. It's about being alert and intentional. This part of a healthy life is the most difficult for most people—and it's often left behind in the attempt at living healthier. But please, stick with it. This is where consistency is particularly important. You have to practice meditating every day for at least six weeks until the process has become second nature to you and you can enjoy its effect. If it helps, begin by practicing in a group or guided by a recording.

I myself find it difficult, every once in a while, to find time for regular meditation. It's important not to see it as an additional task, but as time for yourself, for what's actually important in life. By doing so, the essential spirituality that is connected to meditation becomes vivid. The experience of illness and the limitations of your own corporeality especially are a reminder to dedicate yourself to the exciting question of "Why?" in life.

I meditate while sitting, because lying down I fall asleep too quickly—almost everyone does, and while sleeping is not a bad thing, it isn't meditation. When I meditate depends on my family and work life. In summer, when I wake up earlier, I tend to meditate early in the morning. In winter it's usually in the evening.

I try to integrate exercise into my daily routine: During the week, I ride my bike to work if the weather allows; on weekends I run or walk. At home I practice yoga for a few minutes every day in order to adjust myself internally and externally. I use the step counter on my smartphone, and I recently got a standing desk for my office. Always take the time for these things wherever you can: when watching television, for example, or when "hanging out" in front of the computer. Spend as little time as possible in the car—you can meditate while commuting on the train or the subway.

Mind-body medicine can accomplish much more than just fight stress, even though that is an essential function. It helps us achieve internal freedom. This is hard to describe—you have to experience it, and many of my patients are able to describe their experiences with mind-body medicine rather vividly where dealing with their illnesses and their symptoms is concerned. But it also plays a role in an aging society in general. It's hard for us to face ourselves as aging people, because we always feel younger than we actually are. It's not so much about wrinkles—it's that we yearn for the past, for the feeling of a time when all opportunities were open to us, the energy, the vitality. By using mindfulness or meditation, we can achieve something that is usually lost in the debate about anti-aging: We create a space for mental freedom and timelessness.

A healthy life includes not going to the doctor all that often—as paradoxical as that may sound. This, of course, doesn't mean dealing with serious or indeterminable symptoms by yourself. You do need a doctor to do that. But if you live healthily and utilize naturopathic self-help strategies such as yoga, medicinal herbs, sauna, or cold Scotch hose treatments or moist compresses regularly, you pay more attention to your body and don't rely solely on medications. And that way, you also avoid the negative spiral of symptoms and medications and side effects and further medication and so on. Good medicine supports self-healing processes instead of suppressing them through medication—every dedicated GP knows this. Only those issues that pose actual danger or that cause actual suffering should be treated. In current specialized literature, "choosing wisely" are the keywords here—choosing what actually needs medical treatment by using your common sense. This also means that you are mindful in realizing at what point medical help is necessary instead of trying out different things by experimenting on yourself for too long.

Speaking of "choosing wisely": One thing you can do every day that has a massive influence on your health is the decision about what you eat. Nowadays, even cafeterias usually offer vegetarian menus or salad bars, and you can at least decide what it is you definitely don't want to eat: Reduce your intake of animal protein wherever you can.

Eat as little fast food as possible. Reduce your consumption of alcohol and nicotine (quitting smoking gives you years of additional lifetime!). Avoid products that are polluted with chemicals—be it in their production (pesticides, insecticides, antibiotics) or further processing (additives in convenience products). Turn your back on in-between temptations (snacks)—you'll see how good you feel when you rediscover the natural rhythm of your meals.

But your life shouldn't consist of prohibitions. It's possible to fashion a healthy life in a positive manner—with exceedingly delicious superfoods. These are foodstuffs that contain such large quantities of beneficial substances that they are actually medications, just without the impairing side effects. Unfortunately, the trend is to advertise mainly superfoods that are exotic and have traveled long distances. But most of them can be obtained from local or regional farming, and that way they are controlled and affordable. If you eat only two superfoods from this selection every day, you'll already be doing a lot for your health.

## BERRIES

All types of berries are high in antioxidants. Cranberries prevent inflammations of the bladder. They lower blood pressure in women after menopause and ensure elastic vessel walls. Blueberry juice (not from concentrate) helps with diarrhea and, consumed regularly, protects you from cardiovascular diseases, maybe even from cancer, just like other berries. In instances of macular degeneration, it is speculated that goji berries from China have a special use, because the pigment zeaxanthin that they contain accumulates in the retina and seems to develop a protective effect (incidentally, the same goes for saffron). Berries hardly lose any of their effectiveness after being frozen, but they do when preserved as jam. Even though they contain a lot of fructose, they are generally easily digested.

## FRUITS AND VEGETABLES

These should be organic, seasonal, and ripe. Red and yellow kinds, for example, pumpkin, bell peppers, and tomatoes, contain particularly large amounts of micronutrients. The lycopene they contain, which is only released when they are heated, is healthy for the heart and has many other positive effects. The nutritious yam is probably the reason the inhabitants of the Japanese region of Okinawa reach such an old age. Today it is also cultivated in Italy, Spain, and Portugal. Eat fruits and vegetables as often as you can and ideally whole (for example, a whole orange) instead of in the form of an extract (orange juice). A rich aroma is a better indicator for richness than a shiny outward appearance.

## LEAFY GREENS

Whether it's lettuce, arugula, chard, or spinach—leafy greens are particularly healthy. They contain valuable plant-based nitrate, omega-3 fatty acids, and mineral substances. If you eat leafy greens every day, according to studies, the risk of heart attacks, strokes, and cancer drops by 20 percent.[1] Well then, bye-bye, spinach-phobia! Think of Popeye and put some greens on the table!

## CRUCIFEROUS VEGETABLES

This is another extremely healthy subgroup. It includes broccoli, Brussels sprouts, kale, cress, and arugula—as well as horseradish, mustard, or radishes. They all produce mustard oils to protect themselves from insects and pests. More than one hundred of these oils have already been identified; they are recognizable by their pungent or tangy taste. They kill bacteria and viruses (a concentrated preparation combines cress extract with horseradish extracts, which is very effective in treating sore throats or bladder infections). It's presumed that they can prevent cancer. The mustard oils are stored in the plant as inactive precursors (glucosinolates) because otherwise they would harm the plant itself. When the plant cells are damaged, for example, by the bite of an insect, a compound is created with the enzyme myrosinase, also stored separately in the plant, and thus, the active and highly effective mustard oil is created. Sulforaphane has been researched extensively. It is activated mainly when the vegetable is cut and left to air for about thirty minutes. If you cook it straight away, much of it is lost. That's why frozen cruciferous vegetables are a little less healthy, because they were blanched before being frozen.

## FLAXSEED

The inconspicuous seeds are the superfood among superfoods: They lower cholesterol levels and blood pressure. In the form of gruel, they help treat gastritis and stomach problems. They contain valuable plant-based omega-3 fatty acids in highest concentration, which have an anti-inflammatory effect useful in the treatment of rheumatism or arthrosis (administered by external wraps), for example. Eat shredded flaxseed every day and use flaxseed oil (which must be stored in the refrigerator). For external inflammations, you can even make compresses or prepare baths with flaxseed.

## NUTS

Nuts are very healthy: They are the only form of snacks that don't carry disadvantages. The queen among them is the walnut. It improves blood fat levels, lowers the blood pressure, and counteracts arterial stiffness. Hazelnuts are also healthy, as are almonds (which are actually not a nut, but the drupes of rosaceae, the rose family). Brazil nuts provide a lot of selenium, which is important for the immune system, and they lower cholesterol levels. One or two of them a day are enough, since they also contain methionine, an unhealthy sulfurous amino acid. Unsalted pistachios and peanuts are also very healthy, as they lower heightened blood pressure (though peanuts are actually a legume). The Predimed study has shown that eating 30 grams of mixed nuts every day would be enough to significantly reduce the rate of heart attacks, strokes, and diabetes.

## OLIVE OIL

In our own study we were able to demonstrate that it is particularly the unfiltered, cloudy olive oil that contains many healing substances. Use it to season your pasta, vegetables, or salads—without heating it. For frying and cooking there are cheaper, heat-resistant options available.

## BEANS, PEAS, LENTILS

Legumes contain a lot of healthy plant-based protein. The fact that Latinos have good health outcomes despite eating a lot of fat and sugar (the "Hispanic paradox") is attributed to the fact that they traditionally eat a lot of beans and lentils.[2] Numerous large-scale epidemiologic studies conducted at Harvard University confirm that health increases with the percentage of plant-based proteins we consume.[3] Eat a portion of legumes every day, warm, as a salad or a spread. If the long cooking times bothers you, you can also eat precooked legumes from cans or glasses, but they shouldn't be salted too much. Flatulence can be reduced with the aid of spices (turmeric, pepper, ginger, cinnamon, garlic, and cloves). The more regularly you eat legumes, the less discomfort you experience.

## SPICES

Savory and hot spices in particular contain especially large amounts of phytochemicals in highly concentrated form; they contribute to the color and the intense taste. According to current scientific knowledge, turmeric takes top position.[4] It helps in the treatment of inflammatory bowel diseases and rheumatism, improves blood fat levels, and helps against diabetes. Sprinkle turmeric (or curry) over your meals as often as possible. It does color things pretty strongly—clothing, for example. If you don't like its taste, you can make an exception and resort to extracts from the pharmacy. Ginger and caraway also have positive effects. People who season meals with chiles live longer, a reputable study has shown.[5] According to initial clinical data, saffron (which unfortunately is quite expensive) helps against Alzheimer's disease, depression, and macular degeneration.[6] It's best to mix these spices together—turmeric, for example, is much better absorbed when it's combined with black pepper. And so, an Indian curry is an ideal dish and ensures the absorption of the micronutrients. By the way, onions and garlic are also very healthy; garlic is good for the cardiovascular system, onion for the immune system, possibly even for the prevention of cancer. So, season to your heart's content.

### NATURAL SWEETNESS

Even though we should avoid industrial sugar, we don't have to give up sweet things. Chocolate lowers the blood pressure, widens the vessels, and is anti-inflammatory. It should have a cocoa content of more than 50 percent, but it doesn't have to be the, admittedly, quite tart variety with 80 or 90 percent. Chocolate that contains nuts and almonds is also healthy. Untreated cocoa beans, which are available in many organic supermarkets, have quite an intense taste—try them. Dates and dried figs contain a lot of healthy nutrients and enhance every dessert. Honey contains a lot of mineral substances—and it's anti-inflammatory and antibiotic. That's why, applied externally, it is a very good method to facilitate wound repair. But make sure that it's organically produced.

### WATER

It's not yet been scientifically clarified how much fluid we should consume ideally, or what the optimal fluid requirement is. Currently, the estimation is two to three liters, depending, of course, on outside temperatures and one's activity level. Severe headaches or concentration difficulties often disappear after drinking two to three glasses of water. Mental performance at school improves. Avoid plastic bottles, especially when they are heated, as they contain BPA, which is suspected to cause cancer. Coffee and tea are, despite earlier assumptions, healthy. Coffee helps prevent Parkinson's disease and diabetes and improves liver function—as long as it's unsweetened and no milk is added. (Even soy milk reduces the positive effects.) It only heightens blood pressure temporarily and the slightly diuretic effect that coffee has can be compensated by a glass of water, which in Viennese coffee houses is served along with the coffee as a matter of course. Green tea is equally stimulating and even healthier. Mineral waters rich in bicarbonates counteract an acid-rich diet.

I myself follow a lactovegetarian diet, i.e., with vegetables and a small portion of dairy products, but without eggs. I try to eat two or three of the aforementioned superfoods every day, not as a snack but as part of my meals. (Nuts are the only thing I ever snack on.) For my intermittent fasting, I personally have two variations: If I eat late at night, I don't have breakfast and only drink an espresso with a little almond milk the following morning. If I eat early in the evening, I have some warm porridge with flaxseed (shredded), oatmeal, berries, nuts, and sometimes a little ginger and turmeric (the Ayurvedic kind) for breakfast. In the mornings, I have a whole-body Scotch hose treatment, switching between cold and hot water.

To sum up, these are my recommendations:

- Two filling, solid, meals a day, with no snacks.
- A vegetarian diet wherever possible, with lots of berries and nuts.
- Two superfoods every day, alternating among them, with your meals.
- Daily intermittent fasting (fourteen to sixteen hours of not eating, e.g., if dinner was at 7 p.m., the next meal should be after 11 a.m. the following day).

- One week of therapeutic fasting once or twice a year.
- A cold stimulus every day (whole-body or Scotch hose treatment).
- Practice yoga regularly.
- Meditate daily. (If you can't find thirty minutes, you can also do a "mini" meditation on the train or in the office.)
- Integrate physical activity into your daily routine: Walk places more often, take the stairs, take your bike, go on walks in the woods. Overall, 10,000 steps a day are advisable (about 5 kilometers). For endurance training, 45 minutes three times a week is recommendable.
- Avoid sitting for too long; I recommend a standing desk.
- Get sufficient sleep. (I sleep eight hours every night.)

# CHAPTER ELEVEN

# The Future of Medicine

## *What Needs to Change*

E very day, millions of people take medications that ultimately don't help them, because medicine doesn't work in a way that focuses on the individual enough. The ten most-prescribed drugs in the United States help only one out of four patients in the best-case scenario, and only one out of twenty-five in the worst case. In an article in *Nature*, Nicholas Schork calculated these numbers and spoke about "imprecision medicine."[1] Maybe modern medicine is going to succeed in becoming more precise with the aid of genetics and molecular biology. But it would be sensible to draw upon the experiences of naturopathy, which has always taken an individualized approach.

Today, a considerable number of people are already suffering from chronic diseases by the time they are fifty or sixty years of age. Living longer but simultaneously being sick for longer isn't an appealing perspective. Some illnesses are inevitable—not everything in life can be controlled. But we could do a lot to prevent chronic diseases from developing, and thus enjoy reaching a greater age in good health. But this cannot be achieved without naturopathy. Why?

## HYPOTHESIS 1: DOCTORS SHOULD PREVENT DISEASES
## INSTEAD OF MERELY TREATING THEIR CONSEQUENCES

Without a doubt, most of my colleagues would like to choose this path, but many obstacles, including remuneration, block them from that goal. If a physician motivates someone to give up an unhealthy lifestyle, eat healthy, and get enough physical activity, they should be paid more than someone who performs a bypass surgery ten years later. It's high time for prevention to stop leading a life in the shadows. But many physicians lack the knowledge to do so—modern naturopathy can remedy that.

## HYPOTHESIS 2: NATUROPATHY NEEDS
## TO RECEIVE MORE FUNDING

Modern medicine is relatively young. It has prematurely dismissed centuries-old practical knowledge on how to remain as healthy as possible. Instead, it focuses almost exclusively on the measurability of natural sciences and thus suggests objectivity. But life isn't always objective. Medicine isn't an exact science, either, even though it sometimes creates the impression that it is. Therefore, practical knowledge needs to maintain its place in medicine. It can provide impulses for research, as leeches, bloodletting, and fasting have shown. But naturopathy and integrative medicine clearly also need to examine their therapies scientifically and develop them further. The holistic approach of naturopathy requires elaborate studies, which call for more extensive research funding. The return on investment for scientifically supported naturopathy and its utilization in prevention and the therapy of chronic diseases is undoubtedly given. In the long run, we can't afford to keep treating the incessantly growing number of chronic diseases with ever more surgeries and new, and therefore very expensive, medications.

## HYPOTHESIS 3: MEDICINE CAN DO MORE THAN JUST PRESCRIBE MEDICATIONS

Upon close examination, a large part of the seemingly objective conventional medicine is treading on thin ice—at least in regards to scientific evidence. The power of scientific evidence is often weak. It's also problematic that many doctors and scientists who determine treatment guidelines in the responsible commissions receive money from pharmaceutical companies for research or consulting. Even though they profess their independence, it's just not likely.

Finally, there is the problem of the side effects of medication. If the right drugs have been prescribed for the right indication, side effects must be accepted—because in return, the patient receives relief or a cure. But if medications are prescribed haphazardly and for too long, as is the case in many chronic diseases, the relation between benefit and risk is no longer appropriate.

Many patients instinctively feel a resistance toward medications and refuse to take them, and this insufficient "compliance" holds especially true for major widespread diseases and it carries risks. It's not a rare occurrence that we have to painstakingly convince patients in our naturopathic integrative department that it can be important to take, for example, antirheumatic drugs or to opt for the suggested chemotherapy. This advice is more readily taken from us "naturopaths," maybe because we devote more time to listening to patients. So, we should at least reduce the intake of drugs by supplementing naturopathic methods, if not make them completely redundant if at all possible. Misuse undermines their lifesaving function, as you can see in the example of antibiotics.

Preserving therapies using medicinal plants and preventing them from disappearing due to excessive regulation needs to be another goal. Especially the medicines of traditional healing methods, which often consist of a mixture of active substances, and are blocked on the European market even though they possess enormous potential. Pharmaceutical manufacturers that produce plant-based drugs cannot take out a patent on them and are thus unable to afford the expensive research programs that are increasingly demanded by authorities. That's why there needs to be more funding from independent institutions.

## HYPOTHESIS 4: WITHOUT A HEALTHY DIET, HEALTH IS IMPOSSIBLE

What you eat should always be your individual choice. But the labeling of food often serves to deceive rather than be transparent. The percentage of unhealthy fat and sugar in any food item should be presented in a clear manner. And where nutrition is concerned, it's important that professional recommendations are made independently. Recommendations by federal authorities or expert associations should never fall under the influence of lobby groups, such as the agriculture or food processing industry. It's not right that a population should suffer from a heightened risk of chronic diseases because of these particular interests. Likewise, the content of suspicious environmental chemicals like glyphosate has to be reduced. Animals should no longer be "produced" in mass husbandry, but according to farm animal welfare and housing specifications. Vegetarian or vegan food options should find their way into hospitals, kindergartens, schools, cafeterias, hotels, and restaurants.

## HYPOTHESIS 5: A HEALTHY LIFESTYLE IS A PERSONAL RESPONSIBILITY

Great hope is placed on "wiping out" diseases with the aid of genetic therapy. But this is only going to succeed in very few cases, if only for the reason that most diseases affect multiple genes and take different courses. The genetic material is only to "blame" in 10 or 20 percent of the cases at most.[2] Even if you have "bad" genes, you can significantly reduce your risk of disease by adopting a healthy lifestyle. This even has an influence on our children and grandchildren, as epigenetics shows. The manner in which we live therefore doesn't only concern us: We have a responsibility to our children and grandchildren. And it's not a question of austerity, but of finding a lifestyle that is in harmony with our biology. We must become more sensitive to what is good for us.

## HYPOTHESIS 6: MEDICINE NEEDS TO ENCOURAGE PEOPLE

If we can't drive back chronic diseases, medicine will inevitably become two-tier medicine, because it cannot be financed otherwise. Therefore, we have to succeed in motivating people to lead healthier lives. People want agency, and as patients they should have the right to contribute to their convalescence. The medical system, however, almost completely excludes patients from participating in the process. New keywords like "shared decision making" obscure the fact that all players of the health-care system have more power than the patients themselves: lawmakers, hospitals, health insurance companies, inspectors. This needs to change. Mind-body medicine offers important techniques and practices to enable people to take care of themselves better and especially to reduce stress, which just makes everything even worse.

## HYPOTHESIS 7: "CONVENTIONAL MEDICINE" AND NATUROPATHY BELONG TOGETHER.

"Conventional medicine" needs to start taking naturopathy seriously. That this is beneficial for both sides is shown by the example of the Charité Hospital in Berlin—after all, it is here that half of the German winners of the Nobel Prize for Medicine have worked. With two professorships, modern naturopathy is an important feature of their profile. Different naturopathic schools need to evolve from "eminence" to "evidence," as conventional medicine has already been doing for two decades. Both sides should learn from one another and break fresh ground together.

# Acknowledgments

First, thanks to my wife, Ileni, herself a general practitioner and naturopathic MD, who made valuable daily exchanges on many topics possible and who contributed her practical experiences. For so many evenings and weekends, she had to live with me writing and not always being attentive, and I appreciate the motivating support all the more!

Furthermore, I would like to thank:

The entire team of physicians, therapists, nursing staff, and researchers of naturopathy and other departments at the Immanuel Hospital in Berlin and especially the management team of Dr. Rainer Stange, Dr. Ursula Hackermeier, Dr. Christian Kessler, Dr. Barbara Koch, and Dipl.-Psych. Chris von Scheidt for the fruitful and successful years of cooperation.

The executive board of the Immanuel Hospital in Berlin and the Immanuel Diakonie for the establishment and ongoing support of the department and the center for naturopathy.

The Charité University Hospital in Berlin and its faculty for the integration of naturopathy and integrative medicine into research and teaching, and many colleagues at the Charité Hospital for the numerous instances of exciting research cooperation.

The donors and foundations for their generous funding, which made the research that advanced naturopathy over the last two decades possible in the first place.

The private donors and the members of Nature and Medicine e.V., who are making an important contribution to the research and dissemination of naturopathy with their donations and membership fees.

Prof. Dr. Gustav Dobos and his core team at the Department for Integrative Medicine Naturopathy at the hospitals of Essen-Mitte for the many shared years of inspiring research and practice.

Special thanks to Dr. Petra Thorbrietz, who was able to structure my manuscripts and our conversations due to her great expert knowledge, and who has combined it all into a wonderful text.

And last, but not least: my dear mother, who provided me with the basic trust and who sometimes has to struggle with my nutritional recommendations today.

# Notes

## CHAPTER ONE: THE BASIC PRINCIPLES OF NATUROPATHY

1. Betül Kocaadam and Nevin Şanlier, "Curcumin, an Active Component of Turmeric (Curcuma Longa), and Its Effects on Health," *Critical Reviews in Food Science and Nutrition* 57, no. 13 (2015): 2889–95.
2. Ruchi Badoni Semwal, Deepak Kumar Semwal, Sandra Combrinck, and Alvaro M. Viljoen, "Gingerols and Shogaols: Important Nutraceutical Principles from Ginger," *Phytochemistry* 117 (2015): 554–68.
3. Anne-Fleur Perez, Clément Devic, Catherine Colin, and Nicolas Foray, "Les Faibles Doses De Radiations: Vers Une Nouvelle Lecture De L'évaluation Du Risque?" *Bulletin Du Cancer* 102, no. 6 (2015): 527–38.
4. Thomas Brockow, Andreas Wagner, Annegret Franke, Martin Offenbächer, and Karl L. Resch, "A Randomized Controlled Trial on the Effectiveness of Mild Water-filtered Near Infrared Whole-body Hyperthermia as an Adjunct to a Standard Multimodal Rehabilitation in the Treatment of Fibromyalgia," *The Clinical Journal of Pain* 23, no. 1 (2007): 67–75.
5. Raymond W. Lam, Anthony J. Levitt, Robert D. Levitan, Erin E. Michalak, Amy H. Cheung, Rachel Morehouse, Rajamannar Ramasubbu, Lakshmi N. Yatham, and Edwin M. Tam, "Efficacy of Bright Light Treatment, Fluoxetine, and the Combination in Patients With Nonseasonal Major Depressive Disorder," *JAMA Psychiatry* 73, no. 1 (2016): 56–63.
6. Jörg Reichrath and Knuth Rass, "Ultraviolet Damage, DNA Repair and Vitamin D in Nonmelanoma Skin Cancer and in Malignant Melanoma," in *Sunlight, Vitamin D and Skin Cancer* by Jörg Reichrath (New York: Springer, 2014), 208–33.
7. Asta Juzeniene, Zivile Baturaite, and Johan Moan, "Sun Exposure and Melanomas on Sun-Shielded and Sun-Exposed Body Areas," in *Sunlight, Vitamin D and Skin Cancer* by Jörg Reichrath (New York: Springer, 2014), 375–89.
8. Celia O'Hare, Vincent O'Sullivan, Stephen Flood, and Rose Anne Kenny, "Seasonal and Meteorological Associations with Depressive Symptoms in Older Adults: A Geoepidemiological Study," *Journal of Affective Disorders* 191 (2016): 172–79.
9. Steven R. Feldman, Anthony Liguori, Michael Kucenic, Stephen R. Rapp, Alan B. Fleischer, Wei Lang, and Mandeep Kaur, "Ultraviolet Exposure Is a Reinforcing Stimulus in Frequent Indoor Tanners," *Journal of the American Academy of Dermatology* 51, no. 1 (2004): 45–51.
10. Cedric F. Garland, Frank C. Garland, Edward D. Gorham, Martin Lipkin, Harold Newmark, Sharif B. Mohr, and Michael F. Holick, "The Role of Vitamin D in Cancer Prevention," *American Journal of Public Health* 96, no. 2 (2006): 252–61.

11. David G. Hoel, Marianne Berwick, Frank R. De Gruijl, and Michael F. Holick, "The Risks and Benefits of Sun Exposure 2016," *Dermato-Endocrinology* 8, no. 1 (2016).

12. Rosemary L. Schleicher, Maya R. Sternberg, Anne C. Looker, Elizabeth A. Yetley, David A. Lacher, Christopher T. Sempos, Christine L. Taylor, Ramon A. Durazo-Arvizu, Khin L. Maw, Madhulika Chaudhary-Webb, Clifford L. Johnson, and Christine M. Pfeiffer, "National Estimates of Serum Total 25-Hydroxyvitamin D and Metabolite Concentrations Measured by Liquid Chromatography–Tandem Mass Spectrometry in the US Population during 2007–2010," *The Journal of Nutrition* 146, no. 5 (2016): 1051–61.

13. Hoel et al., "The Risks and Benefits of Sun Exposure 2016."

14. Michael F. Holick, "Vitamin D Deficiency," *New England Journal of Medicine* 357, no. 3 (2007): 266–81.

15. S. De Jong, M. Neeleman, J. J. Luykx, M. J. Ten Berg, E. Strengman, H. H. Den Breeijen, L. C. Stijvers, J. E. Buizer-Voskamp, S. C. Bakker, R. S. Kahn, S. Horvath, W. W. Van Solinge, and R. A. Ophoff, "Seasonal Changes in Gene Expression Represent Cell-type Composition in Whole Blood," *Human Molecular Genetics* 23, no. 10 (2014): 2721–28.

16. De Jong et al., "Seasonal Changes in Gene Expression," 2721–28.

17. Hein A.M. Daanen, and Wouter D. Van Marken Lichtenbelt, "Human Whole Body Cold Adaptation," *Temperature* 3, no. 1 (2016): 104–18.

18. R. Imamura, M. Funatsu, H. Kawachi, and H. Tokura, "Effects of wearing long- and mini-skirts for a year on subcutaneous fat thickness and body circumference," in *Environmental Ergonomics IX*, ed. J. Werner and M. Hexamer (Aachen: Environmental Ergonomics IX, Shaker Verlag, 2000), 315–18.

19. Daanen and Van Marken Lichtenbelt, "Human Whole Body Cold Adaptation."

20. Paul Lee, Sheila Smith, Joyce Linderman, Amber B. Courville, Robert J. Brychta, William Dieckmann, Charlotte D. Werner, Kong Y. Chen, and Francesco S. Celi, "Temperature-Acclimated Brown Adipose Tissue Modulates Insulin Sensitivity in Humans," *Diabetes* 63, no. 11 (2014): 3686–98.

21. Brockow et al., "A Randomized Controlled Trial on the Effectiveness of Mild Water-filtered Near Infrared Whole-body Hyperthermia."

22. Evgenios Agathokleous, Mitsutoshi Kitao, and Edward J. Calabrese, "Environmental Hormesis and Its Fundamental Biological Basis: Rewriting the History of Toxicology," *Environmental Research* 165 (2018): 274–78.

23. V. Calabrese, C. Cornelius, A. Trovato-Salinaro, M. Cambria, M. Locascio, L. Rienzo, D. Condorelli, C. Mancuso, A. De Lorenzo, and E. Calabrese, "The Hormetic Role of Dietary Antioxidants in Free Radical-Related Diseases," *Current Pharmaceutical Design* 16, no. 7 (2010): 877–83.

24. Albrecht Falkenbach, J. Kovacs, A. Franke, K. Jörgens, and K. Ammer, "Radon Therapy for the Treatment of Rheumatic Diseases—Review and Meta-analysis of Controlled Clinical Trials," *Rheumatology International* 25, no. 3 (2003): 205–10.

25. Samuli Rautava, Olli Ruuskanen, Arthur Ouwehand, Seppo Salminen, and Erika Isolauri, "The Hygiene Hypothesis of Atopic Disease—An Extended Version," *Journal of Pediatric Gastroenterology and Nutrition* 38, no. 4 (2004): 378–88.

26. Peter Smith, *Explaining Chaos* (Cambridge: Cambridge University Press, 1999).

27. Richard Friebe, *Hormesis: Das Prinzip Der Widerstandskraft: Wie Stress Und Gift Uns Stärker Machen* (München: Hanser, 2016).

28. Aaron Antonovsky, *Unraveling the Mystery of Health: How People Manage Stress and Stay Well* (San Francisco: Jossey-Bass, 1987).

29. Fabrizio Benedetti, "Placebo Effects: From the Neurobiological Paradigm to Translational Implications," *Neuron* 84, no. 3 (2014): 623–37.

30.  C. Sinke, K. Schmidt, K. Forkmann, and U. Bingel, "Expectation Influences the Inter-ruptive Function of Pain: Behavioural and Neural Findings," *European Journal of Pain* 21, no. 2 (2016): 343–56.

31.  Ted J. Kaptchuk, Elizabeth Friedlander, John M. Kelley, M. Norma Sanchez, Efi Kok-kotou, Joyce P. Singer, Magda Kowalczykowski, Franklin G. Miller, Irving Kirsch, and Anthony J. Lembo, "Placebos without Deception: A Randomized Controlled Trial in Irritable Bowel Syndrome," *PLoS ONE* 5, no. 12 (2010).

32.  Ted J. Kaptchuk, John M. Kelley, Lisa A. Conboy, Roger B. Davis, Catherine E. Kerr, Eric E. Jacobson, Irving Kirsch, Rosa N. Schyner, Bong Hyun Nam, Long T. Nguyen, Min Park, Andrea L. Rivers, Claire Mcmanus, Efi Kokkotou, Douglas A. Drossman, Peter Goldman, and Anthony J. Lembo, "Components of Placebo Effect: Randomised Con-trolled Trial in Patients with Irritable Bowel Syndrome," *BMJ* 336, no. 7651 (2008): 999–1003.

33.  M. Schedlowski, P. Enck, W. Rief, and U. Bingel, "Neuro-Bio-Behavioral Mechanisms of Placebo and Nocebo Responses: Implications for Clinical Trials and Clinical Prac-tice," *Pharmacological Reviews* 67, no. 3 (2015): 697–730.

## CHAPTER TWO: THERAPIES OF ANTIQUITY REDISCOVERED

1.   R. T. Sawyer, *Leech Biology and Behavior* (Oxford: Oxford University Press, 1986).

2.   Sawyer, *Leech Biology and Behavior*.

3.   Andreas Michalsen, Manfred Roth, and Gustav Dobos, *Medicinal Leech Therapy* (Stuttgart: Georg Thieme Verlag, 2007).

4.   "Virchow's Biography," Biography of Rudolf Virchow—Berliner Medizinhistorisches Museum EN, accessed November 2018, https://www.bmm-charite.de/biography-of-rudolf-virchow.html.

5.   William S. Fields, "The History of Leeching and Hirudin," *Pathophysiology of Haemo-stasis and Thrombosis* 21, no. 1 (1991): 3–10.

6.   Sam Schulman, Rebecca J. Beyth, Clive Kearon, and Mark N. Levine, "Hemor-rhagic Complications of Anticoagulant and Thrombolytic Treatment," *Chest* 133, no. 6 (2008).

7.   Ingrid Marty, Veronique Péclat, Gailute Kirdaite, Roberto Salvi, Alexander So, and Nathalie Busso, "Amelioration of Collagen-induced Arthritis by Thrombin Inhibi-tion," *Journal of Clinical Investigation* 107, no. 5 (2001): 631–40.

8.   I. P. Baskova, L. L. Zavalova, A. V. Basanova, S. A. Moshkovskii, and V. G. Zgoda, "Protein Profiling of the Medicinal Leech Salivary Gland Secretion by Proteomic Ana-lytical Methods," *Biochemistry (Moscow)* 69, no. 7 (2004): 770–75.

9.   A. Michalsen, "Effect of Leeches Therapy (Hirudo Medicinalis) in Painful Osteoarthri-tis of the Knee: A Pilot Study," *Annals of the Rheumatic Diseases* 60, no. 10 (2001): 986.

10.  Andreas Michalsen, Stefanie Klotz, Rainer Liedtke, Susanne Moebus, Gunther Spahn, and Gustav J. Dobos, "Effectiveness of Leech Therapy in Osteoarthritis of the Knee: A Randomized, Controlled Trial," *Annals of Internal Medicine* 139, no. 9 (2003): 724–30.

11.  Helen Pilcher, "Stuck on You," *Nature* 432, no. 7013 (2004): 10–11.

12.  Stefan Andereya, Sven Stanzel, Uwe Maus, Ralf Mueller-Rath, Torsten Mumme, Chris-tian H. Siebert, Friedrich Stock, and Ulrich Schneider, "Assessment of Leech Therapy for Knee Osteoarthritis: A Randomized Study." *Acta Orthopaedica* 79, no. 2 (2008): 235–43.

13.  Michalsen et al., *Medicinal Leech Therapy*.

14.   J. Bruce Moseley, Kimberly Omalley, Nancy J. Petersen, Terri J. Menke, Baruch A. Brody, David H. Kuykendall, John C. Hollingsworth, Carol M. Ashton, and Nelda P. Wray, "A Controlled Trial of Arthroscopic Surgery for Osteoarthritis of the Knee," *New England Journal of Medicine* 347, no. 2 (2002): 81–88.

15.   Andreas Michalsen, Rainer Lüdtke, Özgür Cesur, Dani Afra, Frauke Musial, Marcus Baecker, Matthias Fink, and Gustav J. Dobos, "Effectiveness of Leech Therapy in Women with Symptomatic Arthrosis of the First Carpometacarpal Joint: A Randomized Controlled Trial," *Pain* 137, no. 2 (2008): 452–59.

16.   Marcus Bäcker, Rainer Lüdtke, Dani Afra, Özgur Cesur, Jost Langhorst, Matthias Fink, Jürgen Bachmann, Gustav J. Dobos, and Andreas Michalsen, "Effectiveness of Leech Therapy in Chronic Lateral Epicondylitis," *The Clinical Journal of Pain* 27, no. 5 (2011): 442–47.

17.   Christoph-Daniel Hohmann, Rainer Stange, Niko Steckhan, Sibylle Robens, Thomas Ostermann, Arion Paetow, and Andreas Michalsen, "The Effectiveness of Leech Therapy in Chronic Low Back Pain," *Deutsches Äerzteblatt Online*, 2018.

18.   Romy Lauche, Holger Cramer, Jost Langhorst, and Gustav Dobos, "A Systematic Review and Meta-Analysis of Medical Leech Therapy for Osteoarthritis of the Knee," *The Clinical Journal of Pain* 30, no. 1 (2014): 63–72.

19.   Naseem Akhtar Qureshi, Gazzaffi Ibrahim Ali, Tamer Shaban Abushanab, Ahmed Tawfik El-Olemy, Meshari Saleh Alqaed, Ibrahim S. El-Subai, and Abdullah. Al-Bedah, "History of Cupping (Hijama): A Narrative Review of Literature," *Journal of Integrative Medicine* 15, no. 3 (2017): 172–81.

20.   Rainer Lüdtke, Uwe Albrecht, Rainer Stange, and Bernhard Uehleke, "Brachialgia Paraesthetica Nocturna Can Be Relieved by 'Wet Cupping'—Results of a Randomised Pilot Study," *Complementary Therapies in Medicine* 14, no. 4 (2006): 247–53.

21.   Lucy Chen and Andreas Michalsen, "Management of Chronic Pain Using Complementary and Integrative Medicine," *BMJ* 357 (April 2017).

22.   Andreas Michalsen, Silke Bock, Rainer Lüdtke, Thomas Rampp, Marcus Baecker, Jürgen Bachmann, Jost Langhorst, Frauke Musial, and Gustav J. Dobos, "Effects of Traditional Cupping Therapy in Patients With Carpal Tunnel Syndrome: A Randomized Controlled Trial," *The Journal of Pain* 10, no. 6 (2009): 601–8.

23.   Romy Lauche, Jost Langhorst, Gustav J. Dobos, and Holger Cramer, "Clinically Meaningful Differences in Pain, Disability and Quality of Life for Chronic Nonspecific Neck Pain—A Reanalysis of 4 Randomized Controlled Trials of Cupping Therapy," *Complementary Therapies in Medicine* 21, no. 4 (2013): 342–47.

24.   M. Teut, A. Ullmann, M. Ortiz, G. Rotter, S. Binting, M. Cree, F. Lotz, S. Roll, and B. Brinkhaus, "Pulsatile Dry Cupping in Chronic Low Back Pain—a Randomized Three-armed Controlled Clinical Trial," *BMC Complementary and Alternative Medicine* 18, no. 1 (2018).

25.   Michael Teut, Stefan Kaiser, Miriam Ortiz, Stephanie Roll, Sylvia Binting, Stefan N. Willich, and Benno Brinkhaus, "Pulsatile Dry Cupping in Patients with Osteoarthritis of the Knee—a Randomized Controlled Exploratory Trial," *BMC Complementary and Alternative Medicine* 12, no. 1 (2012).

26.   Gerry Greenstone, MD, "The History of Bloodletting," *BCMJ* 52, no. 1 (January, February 2010): 12–14, accessed January 14, 2019, https://www.bcmj.org/premise/history-bloodletting#4.

27.   Jennie Cohen, "A Brief History of Bloodletting," History.com, May 30, 2012, accessed January 14, 2019, https://www.history.com/news/a-brief-history-of-bloodletting.

28.  T. Challoner, C. Briggs, M. W. Rampling, and D. J. Thomas, "A Study of the Haemato-
logical and Haemorheological Consequences of Venesection," *British Journal of Hae-
matology* 62, no. 4 (1986): 671–78.

29.  Jerome L. Sullivan, "Blood Donation May Be Good for the Donor: Iron, Heart Disease,
and Donor Recruitment," *Vox Sanguinis* 61, no. 3 (1991): 161–64.

30.  Sullivan, "Blood Donation May Be Good," 161–64.

31.  Peter Brain and Galenus, *Galen on Bloodletting a Study of the Origins, Development
and Validity of His Opinions, with a Translation of the Three Works* (Cambridge: Cambridge University Press, 1986), xiii, 189.

32.  M. Barenbrock, C. Spieker, K. H. Rahn, and W. Zidek, "Therapeutic Efficiency of Phle-
botomy in Posttransplant Hypertension Associated with Erythrocytosis," *Current
Neurology and Neuroscience Reports* 40, no. 4 (October 1993): 241–43.

33.  Khosrow S. Houschyar, Rainer Lüdtke, Gustav J. Dobos, Ulrich Kalus, Martina
Broecker-Preuss, Thomas Rampp, Benno Brinkhaus, and Andreas Michalsen, "Effects
of Phlebotomy-induced Reduction of Body Iron Stores on Metabolic Syndrome: Results from a Randomized Clinical Trial," *BMC Medicine* 10, no. 1 (2012).

34.  Leo R. Zacharski, Bruce K. Chow, Paula S. Howes, Galina Shamayeva, John A. Baron,
Ronald L. Dalman, David J. Malenka, C. Keith Ozaki, and Philip W. Lavori, "Reduc-
tion of Iron Stores and Cardiovascular Outcomes in Patients With Peripheral Arterial
Disease," *JAMA* 297, no. 6 (2007): 603.

35.  J. T. Salonen, K. Nyyssönen, H. Korpela, J. Tuomilehto, R. Seppänen, and R. Salonen,
"High Stored Iron Levels Are Associated with Excess Risk of Myocardial Infarction in
Eastern Finnish Men," *Circulation* 86, no. 3 (1992): 803–11.

36.  Houschyar et al., "Effects of Phlebotomy-induced Reduction of Body Iron Stores on
Metabolic Syndrome."

37.  Lawrie W. Powell, Rebecca C. Seckington, and Yves Deugnier, "Haemochromatosis,"
*The Lancet* 388, no. 10045 (2016): 706–16.

38.  Powell et al., "Haemochromatosis," 706–16.

39.  J. Scott Gabrielsen, Yan Gao, Judith A. Simcox, Jingyu Huang, David Thorup, Deborah
Jones, Robert C. Cooksey, David Gabrielsen, Ted D. Adams, Steven C. Hunt, Paul N.
Hopkins, William T. Cefalu, and Donald A. Mcclain, "Adipocyte Iron Regulates Adiponectin and Insulin Sensitivity," *Journal of Clinical Investigation* 122, no. 10 (2012):
3529–40.

40.  Gabrielsen et al., "Adipocyte Iron Regulates," 3529–40.

41.  L. R. Zacharski, B. K. Chow, P. S. Howes, G. Shamayeva, J. A. Baron, R. L. Dalman,
D. J. Malenka, C. K. Ozaki, and P. W. Lavori, "Decreased Cancer Risk After Iron Reduc-
tion in Patients With Peripheral Arterial Disease: Results From a Randomized Trial,"
*JNCI Journal of the National Cancer Institute* 100, no. 14 (2008): 996–1002.

42.  Salonen et al., "High Stored Iron Levels Are Associated with Excess Risk of Myocardial
Infarction in Eastern Finnish Men."

43.  Sundrela Kamhieh-Milz, Julian Kamhieh-Milz, Yvonne Tauchmann, Thomas Ostermann, Yatin Shah, Ulrich Kalus, Abdulgabar Salama, and Andreas Michalsen, "Regular Blood Donation May Help in the Management of Hypertension: An Observational
Study on 292 Blood Donors," *Transfusion* 56, no. 3 (2015): 637–44.

44.  Saul A. Villeda, Kristopher E. Plambeck, Jinte Middeldorp, Joseph M. Castellano, Kira
I. Mosher, Jian Luo, Lucas K. Smith, Gregor Bieri, Karin Lin, Daniela Berdnik, Rafael
Wabl, Joe Udeochu, Elizabeth G. Wheatley, Bende Zou, Danielle A. Simmons, Xinmin
S. Xie, Frank M. Longo, and Tony Wyss-Coray, "Young Blood Reverses Age-related

Impairments in Cognitive Function and Synaptic Plasticity in Mice," *Nature Medicine* 20, no. 6 (2014): 659–63.

45. Houschyar et al., "Effects of Phlebotomy-induced Reduction of Body Iron Stores on Metabolic Syndrome."

## CHAPTER THREE: THE HEALING POWER OF WATER

1. Karl Eduard Rothschuh, *Geschichte Der Physiologie* (Berlin: Springer, 1953).
2. Rothschuh, *Geschichte Der Physiologie.*
3. Hindermeyer Jacques, "*Geschichte der physikalischen Therapie und der Rehabilitation,*" in *Illustrierte Geschichte der Medizin* by Richard Toellner (Salzburg: Andreas & Andreas, 1986).
4. Alfred Brauchle and Walter Groh, *Zur Geschichte Der Physiotherapie: Naturheilkunde in Ärztlichen Lebensbildern* (Heidelberg: Haug, 1971).
5. Andreas Michalsen, Rainer Lüdtke, Malte Bühring, Günther Spahn, Jost Langhorst, and Gustav J. Dobos, "Thermal Hydrotherapy Improves Quality of Life and Hemodynamic Function in Patients with Chronic Heart Failure," *American Heart Journal* 146, no. 4 (2003): 728–33.
6. Chuwa Tei, Yutaka Horikiri, Jong-Chun Park, Jin-Won Jeong, Kyoung-Sig Chang, Yoshihumi Toyama, and Nobuyuki Tanaka, "Acute Hemodynamic Improvement by Thermal Vasodilation in Congestive Heart Failure," *Circulation* 91, no. 10 (1995): 2582–90.
7. Kurt Kräuchi, Christian Cajochen, Esther Werth, and Anna Wirz-Justice, "Warm Feet Promote the Rapid Onset of Sleep," *Nature* 401, no. 6748 (1999): 36–37.
8. D. Abeck and Malte Bühring, *Naturheilverfahren Und Unkonventionelle Medizinische Richtungen* (Berlin: Springer, 1992).
9. *Handbuch Der Balneologie Und Medizinischen Klimatologie* (Berlin: Springer, 1998).

## CHAPTER FOUR: THE VALUE OF RESTRAINT

1. "Global Burden of Disease (GBD)," Institute for Health Metrics and Evaluation, December 17, 2018, accessed January 14, 2019, http://www.healthdata.org/gbd.
2. John P. A. Ioannidis, "The Challenge of Reforming Nutritional Epidemiologic Research," *JAMA* 320, no. 10 (2018): 969–70.
3. Randall J. Cohrs, Tyler Martin, Parviz Ghahramani, Luc Bidaut, Paul J. Higgins, and Aamir Shahzad, "Translational Medicine Definition by the European Society for Translational Medicine," *European Journal of Molecular & Clinical Medicine* 2, no. 3 (2014): 86.
4. Otto Buchinger, *Das Heilfasten Und Seine Hilfsmethoden Als Biologischer Weg* (Stuttgart: Hippokrates-Verlag, 1960).
5. Annika Rosengren, Steven Hawken, Stephanie Ôunpuu, Karen Sliwa, Mohammad Zubaid, Wael A. Almahmeed, Kathleen Ngu Blackett, Chitr Sitthi-Amorn, Hiroshi Sato, and Salim Yusuf, "Association of Psychosocial Risk Factors with Risk of Acute Myocardial Infarction in 11 119 Cases and 13 648 Controls from 52 Countries (the INTERHEART Study): Case-control Study," *The Lancet* 364, no. 9438 (2004): 953–62.
6. R. Walford, "Physiologic Changes in Humans Subjected to Severe, Selective Calorie Restriction for Two Years in Biosphere 2: Health, Aging, and Toxicological Perspectives," *Toxicological Sciences* 52, no. 2 (1999): 61–65.

7.  Mark P. Mattson, Valter D. Longo, and Michelle Harvie, "Impact of Intermittent Fast-
     ing on Health and Disease Processes," *Ageing Research Reviews* 39 (2017): 46–58.

8.  Alessio Nencioni, Irene Caffa, Salvatore Cortellino, and Valter D. Longo, "Fasting and
     Cancer: Molecular Mechanisms and Clinical Application," *Nature Reviews Cancer* 18,
     no. 11 (2018): 707–19.

9.  Valter D. Longo and Mark P. Mattson, "Fasting: Molecular Mechanisms and Clinical
     Applications," *Cell Metabolism* 19, no. 2 (2014): 181–92.

10.  Stephan P. Bauersfeld, Christian S. Kessler, Manfred Wischnewsky, Annette Jaensch,
     Nico Steckhan, Rainer Stange, Barbara Kunz, Barbara Brückner, Jalid Sehouli, and An-
     dreas Michalsen, "The Effects of Short-term Fasting on Quality of Life and Tolerance
     to Chemotherapy in Patients with Breast and Ovarian Cancer: A Randomized Cross-
     over Pilot Study," *BMC Cancer* 18, no. 1 (2018): 476.

11.  Stefanie De Groot, Maaike P. G. Vreeswijk, Marij J. P. Welters, Gido Gravesteijn, Jan
     J. W. A. Boei, Anouk Jochems, Daniel Houtsma, Hein Putter, Jacobus J. M. Van Der Ho-
     even, Johan W. R. Nortier, Hanno Pijl, and Judith R. Kroep, "The Effects of Short-term
     Fasting on Tolerance to (neo) Adjuvant Chemotherapy in HER2-negative Breast Can-
     cer Patients: A Randomized Pilot Study," *BMC Cancer* 15, no. 1 (2015).

12.  IARC Working Group on the Evaluation of Carcinogenic Risk to Humans, "Red Meat
     and Processed Meat," *IARC Monographs on the Evaluation of Carcinogenic Risks to
     Humans, No. 114* (Lyon, France: International Agency for Research on Cancer, 2018),
     https://www.ncbi.nlm.nih.gov/books/NBK507971/.

13.  Luigi Fontana and Linda Partridge, "Promoting Health and Longevity through Diet:
     From Model Organisms to Humans," *Cell* 161, no. 1 (2015): 106–18.

14.  Longo and Mattson, "Fasting: Molecular Mechanisms and Clinical Applications."

15.  Longo and Mattson, "Fasting."

16.  Heinz Fahrner, *Fasten Als Therapie* (Stuttgart: Verlag Nicht Ermittelbar, 1991).

17.  Mark P. Mattson, Keelin Moehl, Nathaniel Ghena, Maggie Schmaedick, and Aiwu
     Cheng, "Intermittent Metabolic Switching, Neuroplasticity and Brain Health," *Nature
     Reviews Neuroscience* 19, no. 2 (2018): 63–80.

18.  Mahbubur Rahman, Sajjad Muhammad, Mahtab A. Khan, Hui Chen, Dirk A. Ridder,
     Helge Müller-Fielitz, Barbora Pokorná, Tillman Vollbrandt, Ines Stölting, Roger
     Nadrowitz, Jürgen G. Okun, Stefan Offermanns, and Markus Schwaninger, "The
     β-hydroxybutyrate Receptor HCA2 Activates a Neuroprotective Subset of Macro-
     phages," *Nature Communications* 5, no. 1 (2014): 3944.

19.  Laurence Eyres, Michael F. Eyres, Alexandra Chisholm, and Rachel C. Brown, "Coco-
     nut Oil Consumption and Cardiovascular Risk Factors in Humans," *Nutrition Reviews*
     74, no. 4 (2016): 267–80.

20.  Rafael De Cabo, Didac Carmona-Gutierrez, Michel Bernier, Michael N. Hall, and
     Frank Madeo, "The Search for Antiaging Interventions: From Elixirs to Fasting
     Regimens," *Cell* 157, no. 7 (2014): 1515–26.

21.  Amandine Chaix, Amir Zarrinpar, Phuong Miu, and Satchidananda Panda, "Time-
     Restricted Feeding Is a Preventative and Therapeutic Intervention against Diverse
     Nutritional Challenges," *Cell Metabolism* 20, no. 6 (2014): 991–1005.

22.  Valter D. Longo and Satchidananda Panda, "Fasting, Circadian Rhythms, and Time-
     Restricted Feeding in Healthy Lifespan," *Cell Metabolism* 23, no. 6 (2016): 1048–59.

23.  Frank Madeo, Tobias Eisenberg, Federico Pietrocola, and Guido Kroemer, "Spermi-
     dine in Health and Disease," *Science* 359, no. 6374 (2018).

24.  Carlos López-Otín, Lorenzo Galluzzi, José M. P. Freije, Frank Madeo, and Guido Kro-
     emer, "Metabolic Control of Longevity," *Cell* 166, no. 4 (2016): 802–21.

25. Gerald Huether, Dan Zhou, Sabine Schmidt, Jens Wiltfang, and Eckart Rüther, "Long-term Food Restriction Down-regulates the Density of Serotonin Transporters in the Rat Frontal Cortex," *Biological Psychiatry* 41, no. 12 (1997): 1174–80.

26. L. S. Hermann and M. Iversen, "Death During Therapeutic Starvation," *The Lancet* 292, no. 7561 (1968): 217.

27. A. G. Dulloo and J. P. Montani, "Pathways from Dieting to Weight Regain, to Obesity and to the Metabolic Syndrome: An Overview," *Obesity Reviews* 16 (2015): 1–6.

28. Andreas Michalsen and Chenying Li, "Fasting Therapy for Treating and Preventing Disease—Current State of Evidence," *Forschende Komplementärmedizin / Research in Complementary Medicine* 20, no. 6 (2013): 444–53.

29. Giulia Cesaroni, Francesco Forastiere, Massimo Stafoggia, Zorana J. Andersen, Chiara Badaloni, Rob Beelen, Barbara Caracciolo, Ulf De Faire, Raimund Erbel, Kirsten T. Eriksen, Laura Fratiglioni, Claudia Galassi, Regina Hampel, Margit Heier, Frauke Hennig, Agneta Hilding, Barbara Hoffmann, Danny Houthuijs, Karl-Heinz Jöckel, Michal Korek, Timo Lanki, Karin Leander, Patrik K. E. Magnusson, Enrica Migliore, Caes-Göran Ostenson, Kim Overvad, Nancy L. Pedersen, Juha Pekkanen, Johanna Penell, Göran Pershagen, Andrei Pyko, Ole Raaschou-Nielsen, Andrea Ranzi, Fulvio Ricceri, Veikko Salomaa, Wim Swart, Anu W. Turunen, Paolo Vineis, Gudrun Weinmayr, Kathrin Wolf, Kees De Hoogh, Gerard Hoek, Bert Brunekreef, Annette Peters, and Carlotta Sacerdote, "Long Term Exposure to Ambient Air Pollution and Incidence of Acute Coronary Events: Prospective Cohort Study and Meta-analysis in 11 European Cohorts from the ESCAPE Project," *BMJ*, January 21, 2014, accessed January 14, 2019, https://www.bmj.com/content/348/bmj.f7412.

30. Kristin G. Homme, Janet K. Kern, Boyd E. Haley, David A. Geier, Paul G. King, Lisa K. Sykes, and Mark R. Geier, "New Science Challenges Old Notion That Mercury Dental Amalgam Is Safe," *BioMetals* 27, no. 1 (2014): 19–24.

31. J. S. Lim, H. K. Son, S. K. Park, D. R. Jacobs, and D. H. Lee, "Inverse Associations between Long-term Weight Change and Serum Concentrations of Persistent Organic Pollutants," *International Journal of Obesity* 35, no. 5 (2010): 744–47.

32. Katja Matt, Katharina Burger, Daniel Gebhard, and Jörg Bergemann, "Influence of Calorie Reduction on DNA Repair Capacity of Human Peripheral Blood Mononuclear Cells," *Mechanisms of Ageing and Development* 154 (2016): 24–29.

33. Kristin Prehn, Reiner Jumpertz Von Schwartzenberg, Knut Mai, Ulrike Zeitz, A. Veronica Witte, Dierk Hampel, Anna-Maria Szela, Sonja Fabian, Ulrike Grittner, Joachim Spranger, and Agnes Flöel, "Caloric Restriction in Older Adults—Differential Effects of Weight Loss and Reduced Weight on Brain Structure and Function," *Cerebral Cortex* 27, no. 3 (March 1, 2017): 1765–78.

34. Kenichi Iwashige, Katsuyasu Kouda, Mitsuo Kouda, Kentaro Horiuchi, Masaaki Takahashi, Akira Nagano, Toshiro Tanaka, and Hiroichi Takeuchi, "Calorie Restricted Diet and Urinary Pentosidine in Patients with Rheumatoid Arthritis," *Journal of Physiological Anthropology and Applied Human Science* 23, no. 1 (2004): 19–24.

35. Dr. Somwail Rasla, Memorial Hospital of Alpert Medical School of Brown University in Providence, Rhode Island, American Heart Association, Scientific Sessions 2016, New Orleans, November 12–16, 2016.

36. Andreas Michalsen, Martin K. Kuhlmann, Rainer Lüdtke, Marcus Bäcker, Jost Langhorst, and Gustav J. Dobos, "Prolonged Fasting in Patients with Chronic Pain Syndromes Leads to Late Mood-enhancement Not Related to Weight Loss and Fasting-induced Leptin Depletion," *Nutritional Neuroscience* 9, no. 5–6 (2006): 195–200.

37. Alan C. Goldhamer, Douglas J. Lisle, Peter Sultana, Scott V. Anderson, Banoo Parpia, Barry Hughes, and T. Colin Campbell, "Medically Supervised Water-Only Fasting in the Treatment of Borderline Hypertension," *The Journal of Alternative and Complementary Medicine* 8, no. 5 (2002): 643–50.

38. Alan Goldhamer, Douglas Lisle, Banoo Parpia, Scott V. Anderson, and T. Colin Campbell, "Medically Supervised Water-only Fasting in the Treatment of Hypertension," *Journal of Manipulative and Physiological Therapeutics* 24, no. 5 (2001): 335–39.

39. Sarah Steven, Kieren G. Hollingsworth, Ahmad Al-Mrabeh, Leah Avery, Benjamin Aribisala, Muriel Caslake, and Roy Taylor, "Very Low-Calorie Diet and 6 Months of Weight Stability in Type 2 Diabetes: Pathophysiological Changes in Responders and Nonresponders," *Diabetes Care* 39, no. 5 (2016): 808–15.

40. Jessica Fuhrmeister, Annika Zota, Tjeerd P. Sijmonsma, Oksana Seibert, Şahika Cıngır, Kathrin Schmidt, Nicola Vallon, Roldan M. De Guia, Katharina Niopek, Mauricio Berriel Diaz, Adriano Maida, Matthias Blüher, Jürgen G. Okun, Stephan Herzig, and Adam J. Rose, "Fasting-induced Liver GADD45β Restrains Hepatic Fatty Acid Uptake and Improves Metabolic Health," *EMBO Molecular Medicine* 8, no. 6 (2016): 654–69.

41. Michael Ristow, "Unraveling the Truth About Antioxidants: Mitohormesis Explains ROS-induced Health Benefits," *Nature Medicine* 20, no. 7 (2014): 709–11.

42. L. Göhler, T. Hahnemann, N. Michael, P. Oehme, H.-D. Steglich, E. Conradi, T. Grune, and W. G. Siems, "Reduction of Plasma Catecholamines in Humans during Clinically Controlled Severe Underfeeding," *Preventive Medicine* 30, no. 2 (2000): 95–102.

43. Chia-Wei Cheng, Gregor B. Adams, Laura Perin, Min Wei, Xiaoying Zhou, Ben S. Lam, Stefano Da Sacco, Mario Mirisola, David I. Quinn, Tanya B. Dorff, John J. Kopchick, and Valter D. Longo, "Prolonged Fasting Reduces IGF-1/PKA to Promote Hematopoietic-Stem-Cell-Based Regeneration and Reverse Immunosuppression," *Cell Stem Cell* 14, no. 6 (2014): 810–23.

44. J. S. Bell, J. I. Spencer, R. L. Yates, S. A. Yee, B. M. Jacobs, and G. C. Deluca, "Invited Review: From Nose to Gut—the Role of the Microbiome in Neurological Disease," *Neuropathology and Applied Neurobiology* (October 8, 2018).

45. Lawrence A. David, Corinne F. Maurice, Rachel N. Carmody, David B. Gootenberg, Julie E. Button, Benjamin E. Wolfe, Alisha V. Ling, A. Sloan Devlin, Yug Varma, Michael A. Fischbach, Sudha B. Biddinger, Rachel J. Dutton, and Peter J. Turnbaugh, "Diet Rapidly and Reproducibly Alters the Human Gut Microbiome," *Nature* 505, no. 7484 (2014): 559–64.

46. Xinpu Chen and Sridevi Devaraj, "Gut Microbiome in Obesity, Metabolic Syndrome, and Diabetes," *Current Diabetes Reports* 18, no. 12 (2018): 129.

47. Patrice D. Cani, "Human Gut Microbiome: Hopes, Threats and Promises," *Gut* 67, no. 9 (2018): 1716–25.

48. Cani, "Human Gut Microbiome," 1716–25.

49. Marlene Remely, Berit Hippe, Isabella Geretschlaeger, Sonja Stegmayer, Ingrid Hoefinger, and Alexander Haslberger, "Increased Gut Microbiota Diversity and Abundance of Faecalibacterium Prausnitzii and Akkermansia after Fasting: A Pilot Study," *Wiener Klinische Wochenschrift* 127, no. 9–10 (2015): 394–98.

50. TEDx Talks, "Why Fasting Bolsters Brain Power: Mark Mattson at TEDxJohnsHopkinsUniversity," YouTube, March 18, 2014, accessed January 14, 2019, https://www.youtube.com/watch?v=4UkZAwKoCP8.

51. TEDx Talks, "Why Fasting Bolsters Brain Power."

52. Mark P. Mattson, Keelin Moehl, Nathaniel Ghena, Maggie Schmaedick, and Aiwu Cheng, "Intermittent Metabolic Switching, Neuroplasticity and Brain Health," *Nature Reviews Neuroscience* 19, no. 2 (2018): 63–80.

53. Mattson et al., "Intermittent Metabolic Switching," 63–80.

54. In Young Choi, Laura Piccio, Patra Childress, Bryan Bollman, Arko Ghosh, Sebastian Brandhorst, Jorge Suarez, Andreas Michalsen, Anne H. Cross, Todd E. Morgan, Min Wei, Friedemann Paul, Markus Bock, and Valter D. Longo, "A Diet Mimicking Fasting Promotes Regeneration and Reduces Autoimmunity and Multiple Sclerosis Symptoms," *Cell Reports* 15, no. 10 (2016): 2136–46.

55. A. Michalsen, W. Weidenhammer, D. Melchart, J. Langhorst, J. Saha, and G. Dobos, "Kurzzeitiges Therapeutisches Fasten in Der Behandlung Von Chronischen Schmerz- Und Erschöpfungssyndromen—Verträglichkeit Und Nebenwirkungen Mit Und Ohne Begleitende Mineralstoffergänzung," *Complementary Medicine Research* 9, no. 4 (2002): 221–27.

56. Shubhroz Gill and Satchidananda Panda, "A Smartphone App Reveals Erratic Diurnal Eating Patterns in Humans That Can Be Modulated for Health Benefits," *Cell Metabolism* 22, no. 5 (2015): 789–98.

57. Hana Kahleova, Lenka Belinova, Hana Malinska, Olena Oliyarnyk, Jaroslava Trnovska, Vojtech Skop, Ludmila Kazdova, Monika Dezortova, Milan Hajek, Andrea Tura, Martin Hill, and Terezie Pelikanova, "Erratum To: Eating Two Larger Meals a Day (Breakfast and Lunch) Is More Effective than Six Smaller Meals in a Reduced-energy Regimen for Patients with Type 2 Diabetes: A Randomised Crossover Study," *Diabetologia* 58, no. 1 (2014): 205.

58. Ameneh Madjd, Moira A. Taylor, Alireza Delavari, Reza Malekzadeh, Ian A. Macdonald, and Hamid R. Farshchi, "Beneficial Effect of High Energy Intake at Lunch Rather than Dinner on Weight Loss in Healthy Obese Women in a Weight-loss Program: A Randomized Clinical Trial," *The American Journal of Clinical Nutrition* 104, no. 4 (2016): 982–89.

59. Mark P. Mattson, "Energy Intake and Exercise as Determinants of Brain Health and Vulnerability to Injury and Disease," *Cell Metabolism* 16, no. 6 (2012): 706–22.

60. Tatiana Moro, Grant Tinsley, Antonino Bianco, Giuseppe Marcolin, Quirico Francesco Pacelli, Giuseppe Battaglia, Antonio Palma, Paulo Gentil, Marco Neri, and Antonio Paoli, "Effects of Eight Weeks of Time-restricted Feeding (16/8) on Basal Metabolism, Maximal Strength, Body Composition, Inflammation, and Cardiovascular Risk Factors in Resistance-trained Males," *Journal of Translational Medicine* 14, no. 1 (2016): 290.

61. Catherine R. Marinac, Sandahl H. Nelson, Caitlin I. Breen, Sheri J. Hartman, Loki Natarajan, John P. Pierce, Shirley W. Flatt, Dorothy D. Sears, and Ruth E. Patterson, "Prolonged Nightly Fasting and Breast Cancer Prognosis," *JAMA Oncology* 2, no. 8 (2016): 1049–55.

62. Alessio Nencioni, Irene Caffa, Salvatore Cortellino, and Valter D. Longo, "Fasting and Cancer: Molecular Mechanisms and Clinical Application," *Nature Reviews Cancer* 18, no. 11 (2018): 707–19.

63. Hermann Hesse, *Siddhartha. An Indian Poem: A New Translation by Susan Bernofsky* (New York: The Modern Library, 2008), 54.

## CHAPTER FIVE: THE KEY TO HEALTH

1. "Diet, Nutrition and the Prevention of Chronic Diseases," World Health Organization, October 06, 2014, accessed January 14, 2019, https://www.who.int/dietphysicalactivity /publications/trs916/en/.

2. Cristin E. Kearns, Laura A. Schmidt, and Stanton A. Glantz, "Sugar Industry and Coronary Heart Disease Research," *JAMA Internal Medicine* 176, no. 11 (2016): 1680.

3. Daniel G. Aaron and Michael B. Siegel, "Sponsorship of National Health Organizations by Two Major Soda Companies," *American Journal of Preventive Medicine* 52, no. 1 (2017): 20–30.

4. Michael Greger and Gene Stone, *How Not to Die: Discover the Foods Scientifically Proven to Prevent and Reverse Disease* (New York: Flatiron Books, 2015).

5. Neal D. Barnard, Dreena Burton, and Marilu Henner, *The Cheese Trap: How Breaking a Surprising Addiction Will Help You Lose Weight, Gain Energy, and Get Healthy* (New York: Grand Central Life & Style, 2017).

6. Greger and Stone, *How Not to Die*.

7. Lewis C. Cantley, "Cancer, Metabolism, Fructose, Artificial Sweeteners, and Going Cold Turkey on Sugar," *BMC Biology* 12, no. 1 (2014): 8.

8. "National Center for Health Statistics," Centers for Disease Control and Prevention, May 03, 2017, accessed January 14, 2019, https://www.cdc.gov/nchs/fastats/obesity -overweight.htm.

9. Dean Ornish, Jue Lin, June M. Chan, Elissa Epel, Colleen Kemp, Gerdi Weidner, Ruth Marlin, Steven J. Frenda, Mark Jesus M Magbanua, Jennifer Daubenmier, Ivette Estay, Nancy K. Hills, Nita Chainani-Wu, Peter R. Carroll, and Elizabeth H. Blackburn, "Effect of Comprehensive Lifestyle Changes on Telomerase Activity and Telomere Length in Men with Biopsy-proven Low-risk Prostate Cancer: 5-year Follow-up of a Descriptive Pilot Study," *The Lancet Oncology* 14, no. 11 (2013): 1112–20.

10. Dean Ornish, "Intensive Lifestyle Changes for Reversal of Coronary Heart Disease," *JAMA* 280, no. 23 (1998): 2001–07.

11. Ornish et al., "Effect of Comprehensive Lifestyle Changes on Telomerase Activity and Telomere Length in Men with Biopsy-proven Low-risk Prostate Cancer."

12. Michel de Lorgeril, Patricia Salen, Jean-Louis Martin, Isabelle Monjaud, Jacques Delaye, and Nicole Mamelle, "Mediterranean Diet, Traditional Risk Factors, and the Rate of Cardiovascular Complications After Myocardial Infarction," *Circulation* 99, no. 6 (1999): 779–85.

13. Delfin Rodriguez-Leyva, Wendy Weighell, Andrea L. Edel, Renee Lavallee, Elena Dibrov, Reinhold Pinneker, Thane G. Maddaford, Bram Ramjiawan, Michel Aliani, Randolph Guzman, and Grant N. Pierce, "Potent Antihypertensive Action of Dietary Flaxseed in Hypertensive Patients," *Hypertension* 62, no. 6 (2013): 1081–89.

14. Michael Pollan, *In Defense of Food: An Eater's Manifesto* (London: Penguin Books, 2009).

15. Pollan, *In Defense of Food*.

16. Pollan, *In Defense of Food*.

17. Thomas M. Campbell and T. Colin Campbell, *The China Study: Revised and Expanded Edition* (Dallas: BenBella Books, 2016).

18. Kayo Kurotani, Shamima Akter, Ikuko Kashino, Atsushi Goto, Tetsuya Mizoue, Mitsuhiko Noda, Shizuka Sasazuki, Norie Sawada, and Shoichiro Tsugane, "Quality of Diet and Mortality among Japanese Men and Women: Japan Public Health Center Based Prospective Study," *BMJ 352* (March 2016): i1209.

19. Dan Buettner, *The Blue Zones: Lessons for Living Longer from the People Who've Lived the Longest* (Washington, D.C.: National Geographic, 2008).

20. Ancel Benjamin Keys, *Seven Countries: A Multivariate Analysis of Death and Coronary Heart Disease* (Cambridge, MA: Harvard University Press, 1980).

21. Walter C. Willett, P. J. Skerrett, Edward L. Giovannucci, and Maureen Callahan, *Eat, Drink, and Be Healthy: The Harvard Medical School Guide to Healthy Eating* (New York: Simon & Schuster Source, 2001).

22. R. Estruch, E. Ros, J. Salas-Salvadó, M.-I. Covas, D. Corella, F. Arós, et al., "Primary Prevention of Cardiovascular Disease with a Mediterranean Diet," *New England Journal of Medicine* 368 (2013): 1279–90.

23. Christa B. Hauswirth, Martin R. L. Scheeder, and Jürg H. Beer, "High ω-3 Fatty Acid Content in Alpine Cheese," *Circulation* 109, no. 1 (2004): 103–07.

24. Greger and Stone, *How Not to Die.*

25. Hans Konrad Biesalski, Stephan C. Bischoff, Matthias Pirlich and Arved Weimann, *Ernährungsmedizin: Nach dem Curriculum Ernährungsmedizin der Bundesärztekammer* (Stuttgart: Georg Thieme Verlag, 2018).

26. Dagfinn Aune, Nana Keum, Edward Giovannucci, Lars T. Fadnes, Paolo Boffetta, Darren C. Greenwood, Serena Tonstad, Lars J. Vatten, Elio Riboli, and Teresa Norat, "Whole Grain Consumption and Risk of Cardiovascular Disease, Cancer, and All Cause and Cause Specific Mortality: Systematic Review and Dose-response Meta-analysis of Prospective Studies," *BMJ* (2016): i2716.

27. The Editors of Encyclopaedia Britannica, "John Harvey Kellogg," Encyclopaedia Britannica, December 10, 2018, accessed January 14, 2019, https://www.britannica.com/biography/John-Harvey-Kellogg.

28. Gary Taubes, *Good Calories, Bad Calories: Fats, Carbs, and the Controversial Science of Diet and Health* (New York: Anchor, 2008).

29. Tobias Hoch, Silke Kreitz, Simone Gaffling, Monika Pischetsrieder, and Andreas Hess, "Fat/Carbohydrate Ratio but Not Energy Density Determines Snack Food Intake and Activates Brain Reward Areas," *Scientific Reports* 5, no. 1 (2015).

30. Lewis C. Cantley, "Seeking out the Sweet Spot in Cancer Therapeutics: An Interview with Lewis Cantley," *Disease Models & Mechanisms* 9, no. 9 (2016): 911–16.

31. John Yudkin, *Pure, White, and Deadly: How Sugar Is Killing Us and What We Can Do to Stop It* (New York: Penguin Books, 2013).

32. Robert H. Lustig, *Fat Chance: Beating the Odds against Sugar, Processed Food, Obesity, and Disease* (New York: Plume, 2014).

33. Costas A. Lyssiotis and Lewis C. Cantley. "F Stands for Fructose and Fat," *Nature* 502, no. 7470 (2013): 181–82.

34. T. Jensen, M. F. Abdelmalek, S. Sullivan, K. J. Nadeau, M. Green, C. Roncal, T. Nakagawa, M. Kuwabara, Y. Sato, D. H. Kang, D. R. Tolan, L. G. Sanchez-Lozada, H. R. Rosen, M. A. Lanaspa, A. M. Diehl, and R. J. Johnson, "Fructose and Sugar: A Major Mediator of Non-alcoholic Fatty Liver Disease," Current Neurology and Neuroscience Reports, May 2018, accessed January 14, 2019, https://www.ncbi.nlm.nih.gov/pubmed/29408694.

35. Allison M. Meyers, Devry Mourra, and Jeff A. Beeler, "High Fructose Corn Syrup Induces Metabolic Dysregulation and Altered Dopamine Signaling in the Absence of Obesity," *PLoS One* 12, no. 12 (2017).

36. Martin Raithel, Michael Weidenhiller, Alexander Fritz-Karl Hagel, Urban Hetterich, Markus Friedrich Neurath, and Peter Christopher Konturek, "The Malabsorption of Commonly Occurring Mono and Disaccharides," *Deutsches Aerzteblatt Online*, 2013.

37. Fernando Elijovich, Myron H. Weinberger, Cheryl A. M. Anderson, Lawrence J. Appel, Michael Bursztyn, Nancy R. Cook, Richard A. Dart, Christopher H. Newton-Cheh, Frank M. Sacks, and Cheryl L. Laffer, "Salt Sensitivity of Blood Pressure," *Hypertension* 68, no. 3 (2016): e7–e46.

38. Anna E. Stanhewicz and W. Larry Kenney, "Determinants of Water and Sodium Intake and Output," *Nutrition Reviews* 73, suppl. 2 (2015): 73–82.

39. L. Day, M. A. Augustin, I. L. Batey, and C. W. Wrigley, "Wheat-gluten Uses and Industry Needs," *Trends in Food Science & Technology* 17, no. 2 (2006): 82–90.

40. Martin W. Laass, Roma Schmitz, Holm H. Uhlig, Klaus-Peter Zimmer, Michael Thamm, and Sibylle Koletzko, "The Prevalence of Celiac Disease in Children and Adolescents in Germany," *Deutsches Aerzteblatt Online*, 2015.

41. Alberto Rubio-Tapia, Jonas F. Ludvigsson, Tricia L. Brantner, Joseph A. Murray, and James E. Everhart, "The Prevalence of Celiac Disease in the United States," *The American Journal of Gastroenterology* 107, no. 10 (2012): 1538–44.

42. Imran Pasha, Farhan Saeed, Muhammad Tauseef Sultan, Rizwana Batool, Mahwash Aziz, and Waqas Ahmed, "Wheat Allergy and Intolerence; Recent Updates and Perspectives," *Critical Reviews in Food Science and Nutrition* 56, no. 1 (2013): 13–24.

43. Carlo Catassi, Julio C. Bai, Bruno Bonaz, Gerd Bouma, Antonio Calabrò, Antonio Carroccio, Gemma Castillejo, Carolina Ciacci, Fernanda Cristofori, Jernej Dolinsek, Ruggiero Francavilla, Luca Elli, Peter Green, Wolfgang Holtmeier, Peter Koehler, Sibylle Koletzko, Christof Meinhold, David Sanders, Michael Schumann, Detlef Schuppan, Reiner Ullrich, Andreas Vécsei, Umberto Volta, Victor Zevallos, Anna Sapone, and Alessio Fasano, "Non-Celiac Gluten Sensitivity: The New Frontier of Gluten Related Disorders," MDPI, September 26, 2013, accessed January 14, 2019, https://www.mdpi.com/2072-6643/5/10/3839.

44. Jessica R. Biesiekierski, Evan D. Newnham, Peter M. Irving, Jacqueline S. Barrett, Melissa Haines, James D. Doecke, Susan J. Shepherd, Jane G. Muir, and Peter R. Gibson, "Gluten Causes Gastrointestinal Symptoms in Subjects Without Celiac Disease: A Double-Blind Randomized Placebo-Controlled Trial," *The American Journal of Gastroenterology* 106, no. 3 (2011): 508–14.

45. Patrice D. Cani, "Human Gut Microbiome: Hopes, Threats and Promises," *Gut* 67, no. 9 (2018): 1716–25.

46. Lawrence A. David, Corinne F. Maurice, Rachel N. Carmody, David B. Gootenberg, Julie E. Button, Benjamin E. Wolfe, Alisha V. Ling, A. Sloan Devlin, Yug Varma, Michael A. Fischbach, Sudha B. Biddinger, Rachel J. Dutton, and Peter J. Turnbaugh, "Diet Rapidly and Reproducibly Alters the Human Gut Microbiome," *Nature* 505, no. 7484 (2013): 559–64.

47. W. H. Wilson Tang, Zeneng Wang, Bruce S. Levison, Robert A. Koeth, Earl B. Britt, Xiaoming Fu, Yuping Wu, and Stanley L. Hazen, "Intestinal Microbial Metabolism of Phosphatidylcholine and Cardiovascular Risk," *New England Journal of Medicine* 368, no. 17 (2013): 1575–84.

48. Nicholas F. McMahon, Michael D. Leveritt, and Toby G. Pavey, "The Effect of Dietary Nitrate Supplementation on Endurance Exercise Performance in Healthy Adults: A Systematic Review and Meta-Analysis," *Sports Medicine* 47, no. 4 (2016): 735–56.

49. Andrew R. Coggan, and Linda R. Peterson, "Dietary Nitrate and Skeletal Muscle Contractile Function in Heart Failure," *Current Heart Failure Reports* 13, no. 4 (2016): 158–65.

50. Jonas Esche, Simone Johner, Lijie Shi, Eckhard Schönau, and Thomas Remer,"Urinary Citrate, an Index of Acid-Base Status, Predicts Bone Strength in Youths and Fracture

Risk in Adult Females," *The Journal of Clinical Endocrinology & Metabolism* 101, no. 12 (2016): 4914–21.

51. Jessica C. Kiefte-De Jong, Yanping Li, Mu Chen, Gary C. Curhan, Josiemer Mattei, Vasanti S. Malik, John P. Forman, Oscar H. Franco, and Frank B. Hu, "Diet-dependent Acid Load and Type 2 Diabetes: Pooled Results from Three Prospective Cohort Studies," *Diabetologia* 60, no. 2 (2016): 270–79.

52. Paweena Susantitaphong, Kamal Sewaralthahab, Ethan M. Balk, Bertrand L. Jaber, and Nicolaos E. Madias, "Short- and Long-Term Effects of Alkali Therapy in Chronic Kidney Disease: A Systematic Review," *American Journal of Nephrology* 35, no. 6 (2012): 540–47.

53. K. Michaelsson, A. Wolk, S. Langenskiold, S. Basu, E. Warensjo Lemming, H. Melhus, and L. Byberg, "Milk Intake and Risk of Mortality and Fractures in Women and Men: Cohort Studies," *BMJ* 349 (2014): g6015.

54. Thomas Remer, Triantafillia Dimitriou, and Friedrich Manz, "Dietary Potential Renal Acid Load and Renal Net Acid Excretion in Healthy, Free-living Children and Adolescents," *The American Journal of Clinical Nutrition* 77, no. 5 (2003): 1255–60.

55. Guenther Boden, Carol Homko, Carlos A. Barrero, T. Peter Stein, Xinhua Chen, Peter Cheung, Chiara Fecchio, Sarah Koller, and Salim Merali, "Excessive Caloric Intake Acutely Causes Oxidative Stress, GLUT4 Carbonylation, and Insulin Resistance in Healthy Men," *Science Translational Medicine* 7, no. 304 (2015).

56. S. Steven and R. Taylor, "Restoring Normoglycaemia by Use of a Very Low Calorie Diet in Long- and Short-duration Type 2 Diabetes," *Diabetic Medicine* 32, no. 9 (2015): 1149–55.

57. Andreas Michalsen and Chenying Li, "Fasting Therapy for Treating and Preventing Disease—Current State of Evidence," *Forschende Komplementärmedizin / Research in Complementary Medicine* 20, no. 6 (2013): 444–53.

58. Mary MacVean, "Why Loma Linda Residents Live Longer than the Rest of Us: They Treat the Body like a Temple," *Los Angeles Times,* July 11, 2015, www.latimes.com /health/la-he-blue-zone-loma-linda-20150711-story.html.

59. Gary E. Fraser and David J. Shavlik, "Ten Years of Life," *Archives of Internal Medicine* 161, no. 13 (2001): 1645.

60. K. J. Carpenter, "Protein Requirements of Adults from an Evolutionary Perspective," *The American Journal of Clinical Nutrition* 55, no. 5 (1992): 913–17.

61. Mingyang Song, Teresa T. Fung, Frank B. Hu, Walter C. Willett, Valter D. Longo, Andrew T. Chan, and Edward L. Giovannucci, "Association of Animal and Plant Protein Intake With All-Cause and Cause-Specific Mortality," *JAMA Internal Medicine* 176, no. 10 (2016): 1453–63.

62. Stephen J. Simpson, David G. Le Couteur, David Raubenheimer, Samantha M. Solon-Biet, Gregory J. Cooney, Victoria C. Cogger, and Luigi Fontana, "Dietary Protein, Aging and Nutritional Geometry," *Ageing Research Reviews* 39 (2017): 78–86.

63. Song et al., "Association of Animal and Plant Protein Intake With All-Cause and Cause-Specific Mortality."

64. K. Michaelsson, A. Wolk, S. Langenskiold, S. Basu, E. Warensjo Lemming, H. Melhus, and L. Byberg, "Milk Intake and Risk of Mortality and Fractures in Women and Men: Cohort Studies," *BMJ* 349 (2014): g6015.

65. Diane Feskanich, Heike A. Bischoff-Ferrari, A. Lindsay Frazier, and Walter C. Willett, "Milk Consumption During Teenage Years and Risk of Hip Fractures in Older Adults," *JAMA Pediatrics* 168, no. 1 (2014): 54–60.

66. Greger and Stone, *How Not to Die.*

67. Carrie R. Daniel, Amanda J. Cross, Corinna Koebnick, and Rashmi Sinha, "Trends in Meat Consumption in the USA," *Public Health Nutrition* 14, no. 4 (2010): 575–83.

68. Catey Hill, "This Chart Proves Americans Love Their Meat," MarketWatch, December 01, 2016, accessed January 14, 2019, https://www.marketwatch.com/story/this-chart -proves-americans-love-their-meat-2016-08-15.

69. Erich Rauch, *Die Darmreinigung Nach Dr. Med. F.X. Mayr: Wie Sie Richtig Entschlacken, Entgiften Und Entsäuern* (Heidelberg: Haug, 2001).

70. Bonnie L. Beezhold and Carol S. Johnston, "Restriction of Meat, Fish, and Poultry in Omnivores Improves Mood: A Pilot Randomized Controlled Trial," *Nutrition Journal* 11, no. 1 (2012): 9.

71. Shuang Tian, Qian Xu, Ruyue Jiang, Tianshu Han, Changhao Sun, and Lixin Na, "Dietary Protein Consumption and the Risk of Type 2 Diabetes: A Systematic Review and Meta-Analysis of Cohort Studies," *Nutrients* 9, no. 9 (2017): 982.

72. W. H. Wilson Tang, Zeneng Wang, Bruce S. Levison, Robert A. Koeth, Earl B. Britt, Xiaoming Fu, Yuping Wu, and Stanley L. Hazen, "Intestinal Microbial Metabolism of Phosphatidylcholine and Cardiovascular Risk," *New England Journal of Medicine* 368, no. 17 (2013): 1575–84.

73. Anahad O'Connor, "Advice from a Vegan Cardiologist," *The New York Times Well* blog, August 6, 2014, https://well.blogs.nytimes.com/2014/08/06/advice-from-a-vegan -cardiologist/.

74. David J. A. Jenkins, "Effects of a Dietary Portfolio of Cholesterol-Lowering Foods vs Lovastatin on Serum Lipids and C-Reactive Protein," *JAMA* 290, no. 4 (2003): 502.

75. Jenkins, "Effects of a Dietary Portfolio of Cholesterol-Lowering Foods," 502.

76. Beth A. Taylor and Paul D. Thompson, "Statin-Associated Muscle Disease: Advances in Diagnosis and Management," *Neurotherapeutics* 15, no. 4 (2018): 1006–17.

77. Takehiro Sugiyama, Yusuke Tsugawa, Chi-Hong Tseng, Yasuki Kobayashi, and Martin F. Shapiro, "Different Time Trends of Caloric and Fat Intake Between Statin Users and Nonusers Among US Adults," *JAMA Internal Medicine* 174, no. 7 (2014): 1038.

78. Greger and Stone, *How Not to Die.*

79. Vesanto Melina, Winston Craig, and Susan Levin, "Position of the Academy of Nutrition and Dietetics: Vegetarian Diets." *Journal of the Academy of Nutrition and Dietetics* 116, no. 12 (2016): 1970–80.

80. Harald Lemke, *Ethik des Essens. Eine Einführung in die Gastrosophie* (Berlin: Akademie Verlag, 2007).

## CHAPTER SIX: STAGNATION IS CAUSE FOR ILLNESS

1. Karl Ed. Rothschuh, "Ernst Schweninger (1850–1924) Zu Seinem Leben Und Wirken: Ergänzungen, Korrekturen," *Medizinhistorisches Journal* 19, no. 3 (1984): 250–58.

2. Siri Kvam, Catrine Lykkedrang Kleppe, Inger Hilde Nordhus, and Anders Hovland, "Exercise as a Treatment for Depression: A Meta-analysis," *Journal of Affective Disorders* 202 (2016): 67–86.

3. Hmwe H. Kyu, Victoria F. Bachman, Lily T. Alexander, John Everett Mumford, Ashkan Afshin, Kara Estep, J. Lennert Veerman, Kristen Delwiche, Marissa L. Iannarone, Madeline L. Moyer, Kelly Cercy, Theo Vos, Christopher J L Murray, and Mohammad H. Forouzanfar, "Physical Activity and Risk of Breast Cancer, Colon Cancer, Diabetes, Ischemic Heart Disease, and Ischemic Stroke Events: Systematic Review and

Dose-response Meta-analysis for the Global Burden of Disease Study 2013," *BMJ* 354 (2016): i3857.

4. Kyu et al., "Physical Activity and Risk."

5. Roy J. Shephard, "Physical Activity and Prostate Cancer: An Updated Review," *Sports Medicine* 47, no. 6 (2016): 1055–73.

6. Q. Li, Kanehisa Morimoto, M. Kobayashi, Hirofumi Inagaki, M. Katsumata, Y. Hirata, K. Hirata, T. Shimizu, Y. J. Li, Y. Wakayama, T. Kawada, Tatsuro Ohira, Norimasa Takayama, Takahide Kagawa, and Yoshifumi Miyazaki, "A Forest Bathing Trip Increases Human Natural Killer Activity and Expression of Anti-cancer Proteins in Female Subjects," *Journal of Biological Regulators and Homeostatic Agents* 22, no. 1 (2008): 45–55.

7. J. Lee, B. J. Park, Y. Tsunetsugu, T. Ohira, T. Kagawa, and Y. Miyazaki, "Effect of Forest Bathing on Physiological and Psychological Responses in Young Japanese Male Subjects," *Public Health* 125, no. 2 (2011): 93–100.

8. R. Ulrich, "View through a Window May Influence Recovery from Surgery," *Science* 224, no. 4647 (1984): 420.

9. Diana E. Bowler, Lisette M. Buyung-Ali, Teri M. Knight, and Andrew S. Pullin, "A Systematic Review of Evidence for the Added Benefits to Health of Exposure to Natural Environments," *BMC Public Health* 10, no. 1 (2010).

10. Nadja Lejtzén, Jan Sundquist, Kristina Sundquist, and Xinjun Li, "Depression and Anxiety in Swedish Primary Health Care: Prevalence, Incidence, and Risk Factors," *European Archives of Psychiatry and Clinical Neuroscience* 264, no. 3 (2013): 235–45.

11. Gregory N. Bratman, J. Paul Hamilton, Kevin S. Hahn, Gretchen C. Daily, and James J. Gross, "Nature Experience Reduces Rumination and Subgenual Prefrontal Cortex Activation," *Proceedings of the National Academy of Sciences* 112, no. 28 (2015): 8567–72.

12. Danielle F. Shanahan, Robert Bush, Kevin J. Gaston, Brenda B. Lin, Julie Dean, Elizabeth Barber, and Richard A. Fuller, "Health Benefits from Nature Experiences Depend on Dose," *Scientific Reports* 6, no. 1 (2016).

13. Chorong Song, Harumi Ikei, and Yoshifumi Miyazaki, "Physiological Effects of Visual Stimulation with Forest Imagery," *International Journal of Environmental Research and Public Health* 15, no. 2 (2018): 213.

14. Nancy Humpel, Neville Owen, Don Iverson, Eva Leslie, and Adrian Bauman, "Perceived Environment Attributes, Residential Location, and Walking for Particular Purposes," *American Journal of Preventive Medicine* 26, no. 2 (2004): 119–25.

15. Kyu et al., "Physical Activity and Risk of Breast Cancer, Colon Cancer, Diabetes, Ischemic Heart Disease, and Ischemic Stroke Events."

16. Christian M. Werner, Anne Hecksteden, Arne Morsch, Joachim Zundler, Melissa Wegmann, Jürgen Kratzsch, Joachim Thiery, Mathias Hohl, Jörg Thomas Bittenbring, Frank Neumann, Michael Böhm, Tim Meyer, and Ulrich Laufs, "Differential Effects of Endurance, Interval, and Resistance Training on Telomerase Activity and Telomere Length in a Randomized, Controlled Study," *European Heart Journal* 40, no. 1 (January 1, 2019): 34–46.

17. Jan Wilke, Robert Schleip, Werner Klingler, and Carla Stecco, "The Lumbodorsal Fascia as a Potential Source of Low Back Pain: A Narrative Review," *BioMed Research International* 2017 (2017): 1–6.

18. Rainer Lüdtke, Uwe Albrecht, Rainer Stange, and Bernhard Uehleke, "Brachialgia Paraesthetica Nocturna Can Be Relieved by 'Wet Cupping'—Results of a Randomised Pilot Study," *Complementary Therapies in Medicine* 14, no. 4 (2006): 247–53.

19. Joseph Henson, David W. Dunstan, Melanie J. Davies, and Thomas Yates, "Sedentary Behaviour as a New Behavioural Target in the Prevention and Treatment of Type 2 Diabetes," *Diabetes/Metabolism Research and Reviews* 32 (2016): 213–20.

## CHAPTER SEVEN: YOGA, MEDITATION, AND MINDFULNESS

1. Mika Kivimäki, Markus Jokela, Solja T. Nyberg, Archana Singh-Manoux, Eleonor I. Fransson, Lars Alfredsson, Jakob B. Bjorner, Marianne Borritz, Hermann Burr, Annalisa Casini, Els Clays, Dirk De Bacquer, Nico Dragano, Raimund Erbel, Goedele A. Geuskens, Mark Hamer, Wendela E. Hooftman, Irene L. Houtman, Karl-Heinz Jöckel, France Kittel, Anders Knutsson, Markku Koskenvuo, Thorsten Lunau, Ida E H Madsen, Martin L. Nielsen, Maria Nordin, Tuula Oksanen, Jan H. Pejtersen, Jaana Pentti, Reiner Rugulies, Paula Salo, Martin J. Shipley, Johannes Siegrist, Andrew Steptoe, Sakari B. Suominen, Töres Theorell, Jussi Vahtera, Peter J M Westerholm, Hugo Westerlund, Dermot Oreilly, Meena Kumari, G. David Batty, Jane E. Ferrie, and Marianna Virtanen, "Long Working Hours and Risk of Coronary Heart Disease and Stroke: A Systematic Review and Meta-Analysis of Published and Unpublished Data for 603 838 Individuals," *The Lancet* 386, no. 10005 (2015): 1739–46.
2. Maurice M. Ohayon, "Epidemiology of Insomnia: What We Know and What We Still Need to Learn," *Sleep Medicine Reviews* 6, no. 2 (2002): 97–111.
3. M. A. Killingsworth and D. T. Gilbert, "A Wandering Mind Is an Unhappy Mind," *Science* 330, no. 6006 (2010): 932.
4. Tetsuya Nakazawa, Yasushi Okubo, Yasushi Suwazono, Etsuko Kobayashi, Shingo Komine, Norihisa Kato, and Koji Nogawa, "Association between Duration of Daily VDT Use and Subjective Symptoms," *American Journal of Industrial Medicine* 42, no. 5 (2002): 421–26.
5. Stefan Brunnhuber, *Die Kunst der Transformation: Wie wir lernen, die Welt zu verändern* (N.P.: Verlag Herder, 2016).
6. Andrew Lepp, Jacob E. Barkley, and Aryn C. Karpinski, "The Relationship between Cell Phone Use, Academic Performance, Anxiety, and Satisfaction with Life in College Students," *Computers in Human Behavior* 31 (2014): 343–50.
7. Lee Rainie, Kathryn Zickuhr, Lee Rainie, and Kathryn Zickuhr, "Americans' Views on Mobile Etiquette," Pew Research Center: Internet, Science & Tech, January 03, 2018, accessed January 23, 2019, http://www.pewinternet.org/2015/08/26/americans-views-on-mobile-etiquette/.
8. Firdaus S. Dhabhar, "Effects of Stress on Immune Function: The Good, the Bad, and the Beautiful," *Immunologic Research* 58, no. 2–3 (2014): 193–210.
9. Dhabhar, "Effects of Stress on Immune Function," 193–210.
10. Richard J. Davidson, Jon Kabat-Zinn, Jessica Schumacher, Melissa Rosenkranz, Daniel Muller, Saki F. Santorelli, Ferris Urbanowski, Anne Harrington, Katherine Bonus, and John F. Sheridan, "Alterations in Brain and Immune Function Produced by Mindfulness Meditation," *Psychosomatic Medicine* 65, no. 4 (2003): 564–70.
11. Firdaus S. Dhabhar, "The Short-term Stress Response—Mother Nature's Mechanism for Enhancing Protection and Performance under Conditions of Threat, Challenge, and Opportunity," *Frontiers in Neuroendocrinology* 49 (2018): 175–92.
12. Shira Meir Drexler and Oliver T. Wolf, "The Role of Glucocorticoids in Emotional Memory Reconsolidation," *Neurobiology of Learning and Memory* 142 (2017): 126–34.

13. Abiola Keller, Kristin Litzelman, Lauren E. Wisk, Torsheika Maddox, Erika Rose Cheng, Paul D. Creswell, and Whitney P. Witt, "Does the Perception That Stress Affects Health Matter? The Association with Health and Mortality," *Health Psychology* 31, no. 5 (2012): 677–84.

14. Brunnhuber, *Die Kunst der Transformation.*

15. Annika Rosengren, Steven Hawken, Stephanie Ôunpuu, Karen Sliwa, Mohammad Zubaid, Wael A. Almahmeed, Kathleen Ngu Blackett, Chitr Sitthi-Amorn, Hiroshi Sato, and Salim Yusuf, "Association of Psychosocial Risk Factors with Risk of Acute Myocardial Infarction in 11 119 Cases and 13 648 Controls from 52 Countries (the INTERHEART Study): Case-control Study," *The Lancet* 364, no. 9438 (2004): 953–62.

16. Hermann Nabi, Mika Kivimäki, G. David Batty, Martin J. Shipley, Annie Britton, Eric J. Brunner, Jussi Vahtera, Cédric Lemogne, Alexis Elbaz, and Archana Singh-Manoux, "Increased Risk of Coronary Heart Disease among Individuals Reporting Adverse Impact of Stress on Their Health: The Whitehall II Prospective Cohort Study," *European Heart Journal* 34, no. 34 (2013): 2697–705.

17. Shwetha Nair, Mark Sagar, John Sollers, Nathan Consedine, and Elizabeth Broadbent, "Do Slumped and Upright Postures Affect Stress Responses? A Randomized Trial," *Health Psychology* 34, no. 6 (2015): 632–41.

18. Beatrice Kennedy, Fang Fang, Unnur Valdimarsdóttir, Ruzan Udumyan, Scott Montgomery, and Katja Fall, "Stress Resilience and Cancer Risk: A Nationwide Cohort Study," *Journal of Epidemiology and Community Health* 71, no. 10 (2017): 947–53.

19. Pi-Chu Lin, "An Evaluation of the Effectiveness of Relaxation Therapy for Patients Receiving Joint Replacement Surgery," *Journal of Clinical Nursing* 21, no. 5–6 (2011): 601–08.

20. Galina Kipnis, Nili Tabak, and Silvia Koton, "Background Music Playback in the Preoperative Setting: Does It Reduce the Level of Preoperative Anxiety Among Candidates for Elective Surgery?" *Journal of PeriAnesthesia Nursing* 31, no. 3 (2016): 209–16.

21. Joke Bradt, Cheryl Dileo, and Minjung Shim, "Music Interventions for Preoperative Anxiety," *Cochrane Database of Systematic Reviews* 6 (June 2013).

22. Herbert Benson and Miriam Z. Klipper, *The Relaxation Response* (New York: HarperTorch, 2000).

23. Benson and Klipper, *The Relaxation Response.*

24. A. Michalsen, P. Grossman, A. Acil, J. Langhorst, R. Lüdtke, T. Esch, G. B. Stefano, and G. J. Dobos, "Rapid Stress Reduction and Anxiolysis among Distressed Women as a Consequence of a Three-Month Intensive Yoga Program," *Medical Science Monitor* 11 (2005).

25. Andreas Michalsen, Michael Jeitler, Stefan Brunnhuber, Rainer Lüdtke, Arndt Büssing, Frauke Musial, Gustav Dobos, and Christian Kessler, "Iyengar Yoga for Distressed Women: A 3-Armed Randomized Controlled Trial," *Evidence-Based Complementary and Alternative Medicine* (2012): 1–9.

26. Sat Bir Singh Khalsa, Lorenzo Cohen, Timothy McCall, and Shirley Telles, *The Principles and Practice of Yoga in Health Care* (Edinburgh: Handspring Publishing, 2016).

27. Andreas Michalsen, Hermann Traitteur, Rainer Lüdtke, Stefan Brunnhuber, Larissa Meier, Michael Jeitler, Arndt Büssing, and Christian Kessler, "Yoga for Chronic Neck Pain: A Pilot Randomized Controlled Clinical Trial," *The Journal of Pain* 13, no. 11 (2012): 1122–30.

28. Dania Schumann, Dennis Anheyer, Romy Lauche, Gustav Dobos, Jost Langhorst, and Holger Cramer, "Effect of Yoga in the Therapy of Irritable Bowel Syndrome: A Systematic Review," *Clinical Gastroenterology and Hepatology* 14, no. 12 (2016): 1720–31.

29.  Janice K. Kiecolt-Glaser, Jeanette M. Bennett, Rebecca Andridge, Juan Peng, Charles L. Shapiro, William B. Malarkey, Charles F. Emery, Rachel Layman, Ewa E. Mrozek, and Ronald Glaser, "Yoga's Impact on Inflammation, Mood, and Fatigue in Breast Cancer Survivors: A Randomized Controlled Trial," *Journal of Clinical Oncology* 32, no. 10 (2014): 1040–49.

30.  Tom Hendriks, Joop De Jong, and Holger Cramer. "The Effects of Yoga on Positive Mental Health Among Healthy Adults: A Systematic Review and Meta-Analysis," *The Journal of Alternative and Complementary Medicine* 23, no. 7 (2017): 505–17.

31.  Holger Cramer, Jost Langhorst, Gustav Dobos, and Romy Lauche, "Yoga for Metabolic Syndrome: A Systematic Review and Meta-analysis," *European Journal of Preventive Cardiology* 23, no. 18 (2016): 1982–93.

32.  Paul Posadzki, Holger Cramer, Adrian Kuzdzal, Myeong Soo Lee, and Edzard Ernst, "Yoga for Hypertension: A Systematic Review of Randomized Clinical Trials," *Complementary Therapies in Medicine* 22, no. 3 (2014): 511–22.

33.  Karen J. Sherman, "A Randomized Trial Comparing Yoga, Stretching, and a Self-care Book for Chronic Low Back Pain," *Archives of Internal Medicine* 171, no. 22 (2011): 2019–26.

34.  Karen J. Sherman, Daniel C. Cherkin, Janet Erro, Diana L. Miglioretti, and Richard A. Deyo, "Comparing Yoga, Exercise, and a Self-Care Book for Chronic Low Back Pain," *Annals of Internal Medicine* 143, no. 12 (2005): 849–56.

35.  Khalsa et al., *Principles and Practice of Yoga in Health Care.*

36.  P. Barthel, R. Wensel, A. Bauer, A. Muller, P. Wolf, K. Ulm, K. M. Huster, D. P. Francis, M. Malik, and G. Schmidt, "Respiratory Rate Predicts Outcome after Acute Myocardial Infarction: A Prospective Cohort Study," *European Heart Journal* 34, no. 22 (2012): 1644–50.

37.  Benson and Klipper, *The Relaxation Response.*

38.  Paul Grossman, Ludger Niemann, Stefan Schmidt, and Harald Walach, "Mindfulness-based Stress Reduction and Health Benefits," *Journal of Psychosomatic Research* 57, no. 1 (2004): 35–43.

39.  Grossman et al., "Mindfulness-based Stress Reduction and Health Benefits," 35–43.

40.  Jenny Gu, Clara Strauss, Rod Bond, and Kate Cavanagh, "How Do Mindfulness-based Cognitive Therapy and Mindfulness-based Stress Reduction Improve Mental Health and Wellbeing? A Systematic Review and Meta-analysis of Mediation Studies," *Clinical Psychology Review* 37 (2015): 1–12.

41.  David W. Orme-Johnson, Robert H. Schneider, Young D. Son, Sanford Nidich, and Zang-Hee Cho, "Neuroimaging of Meditation's Effect on Brain Reactivity to Pain," *NeuroReport* 17, no. 12 (2006): 1359–63.

42.  Benson and Klipper, *The Relaxation Response.*

43.  Tonya L. Jacobs, Elissa S. Epel, Jue Lin, Elizabeth H. Blackburn, Owen M. Wolkowitz, David A. Bridwell, Anthony P. Zanesco, Stephen R. Aichele, Baljinder K. Sahdra, Katherine A. Maclean, Brandon G. King, Phillip R. Shaver, Erika L. Rosenberg, Emilio Ferrer, B. Alan Wallace, and Clifford D. Saron, "Intensive Meditation Training, Immune Cell Telomerase Activity, and Psychological Mediators," *Psychoneuroendocrinology* 36, no. 5 (2011): 664–81.

44.  Sara W. Lazar, Catherine E. Kerr, Rachel H. Wasserman, Jeremy R. Gray, Douglas N. Greve, Michael T. Treadway, Metta Mcgarvey, Brian T. Quinn, Jeffery A. Dusek, Herbert Benson, Scott L. Rauch, Christopher I. Moore, and Bruce Fischl, "Meditation Experience Is Associated with Increased Cortical Thickness," *NeuroReport* 16, no. 17 (2005): 1893–97.

45. J. W. Anderson, C. Liu, and R. J. Kryscio, "Blood Pressure Response to Transcendental Meditation: A Meta-analysis," *American Journal of Hypertension* 21, no. 3 (2008): 310–16.

46. Rajinder Singh, *Meditation as Medication for the Soul* (Lisle, IL: Radiance Publishers, 2012).

47. Luciano Bernardi, Joanna Wdowczyk-Szulc, Cinzia Valenti, Stefano Castoldi, Claudio Passino, Giammario Spadacini, and Peter Sleight, "Effects of Controlled Breathing, Mental Activity and Mental Stress with or without Verbalization on Heart Rate Variability," *Journal of the American College of Cardiology* 35, no. 6 (2000): 1462–69.

48. Shanshan Li, Meir J. Stampfer, David R. Williams, and Tyler J. Vanderweele, "Association of Religious Service Attendance With Mortality Among Women," *JAMA Internal Medicine* 176, no. 6 (2016): 777–85.

## CHAPTER EIGHT: GLOBAL MEDICINES

1. Paul U. Unschuld, *Traditionelle Chinesische Medizin* (München: Beck, 2013).

2. Peter C. Gøtzsche, Richard Smith, and Drummond Rennie, *Deadly Medicines and Organised Crime: How Big Pharma Has Corrupted Healthcare* (London: Radcliffe Publishing, 2013).

3. M. Burnier, "Drug Adherence in Hypertension," *Pharmacological Research* 125 (2017): 142–49.

4. Ajda Ota and Nataša P. Ulrih, "An Overview of Herbal Products and Secondary Metabolites Used for Management of Type Two Diabetes," *Frontiers in Pharmacology* 8 (2017): 436.

5. Helen Tremlett, Kylynda C. Bauer, Silke Appel-Cresswell, Brett B. Finlay, and Emmanuelle Waubant, "The Gut Microbiome in Human Neurological Disease: A Review," *Annals of Neurology* 81, no. 3 (2017): 369–82.

6. Daniel Furst, Manorama M. Venkatraman, Mary McGann, Ram Manohar, Cathryn Booth-LaForce, Reshmi Pushpan, P. G. Sekar, K. G. Raveendran, Anita Mahapatra, Jidesh Gopinath, and P. R. Krishna Kumar, "Double-Blind, Randomized, Controlled, Pilot Study Comparing Classic Ayurvedic Medicine, Methotrexate, and Their Combination in Rheumatoid Arthritis," *Journal of Clinical Rheumatology* 17, no. 4 (2011): 185–92.

7. Shanshan Li, Meir J. Stampfer, David R. Williams, and Tyler J. Vanderweele, "Association of Religious Service Attendance with Mortality Among Women," *JAMA Internal Medicine* 176, no. 6 (2016): 777–85.

8. Tyler J. Vanderweele, Jeffrey Yu, Yvette C. Cozier, Lauren Wise, M. Austin Argentieri, Lynn Rosenberg, Julie R. Palmer, and Alexandra E. Shields, "Attendance at Religious Services, Prayer, Religious Coping, and Religious/Spiritual Identity as Predictors of All-Cause Mortality in the Black Women's Health Study," *American Journal of Epidemiology* 185, no. 7 (2017): 515–22.

9. William C. Stewart, Michelle P. Adams, Jeanette A. Stewart, and Lindsay A. Nelson, "Review of Clinical Medicine and Religious Practice," *Journal of Religion and Health* 52, no. 1 (2012): 91–106.

10. Claudia M. Witt, Susanne Jena, Benno Brinkhaus, Bodo Liecker, Karl Wegscheider, and Stefan N. Willich, "Acupuncture in Patients with Osteoarthritis of the Knee or Hip: A Randomized, Controlled Trial with an Additional Nonrandomized Arm," *Arthritis & Rheumatism* 54, no. 11 (2006): 3485–93.

11. Claudia M. Witt, Susanne Jena, Benno Brinkhaus, Bodo Liecker, Karl Wegscheider, and Stefan N. Willich, "Acupuncture for Patients with Chronic Neck Pain," *Pain* 125, no. 1 (2006): 98–106.

12. B. Brinkhaus, "Acupuncture in Patients With Chronic Low Back Pain: A Randomized Controlled Trial," *Archives of Internal Medicine* 166, no. 4 (2006): 450–57.

13. Claudia Witt, B. Brinkhaus, Susanne Jena, K. Linde, A. Streng, Stefan Wagenpfeil, Josef Hummelsberger, H. U. Walther, Dieter Melchart, and S. N. Willich, "Acupuncture in Patients with Osteoarthritis of the Knee: A Randomised Trial," *Lancet* 366, no. 9480 (July 2005): 136–43.

14. Andrew J. Vickers, Emily A. Vertosick, George Lewith, Hugh Macpherson, Nadine E. Foster, Karen J. Sherman, Dominik Irnich, Claudia M. Witt, and Klaus Linde, "Acupuncture for Chronic Pain: Update of an Individual Patient Data Meta-Analysis," *The Journal of Pain* 19, no. 5 (2018): 455–74.

15. Benno Brinkhaus, Miriam Ortiz, Claudia M. Witt, S. Roll, Klaus Linde, Florian Pfab, Bodo Niggemann, Josef Hummelsberger, András Treszl, Johannes Hofaker Ring, Torsten Zuberbier, Karl Wegscheider, and Stefan N. Willich, "Acupuncture in Patients with Seasonal Allergic Rhinitis: A Randomized Trial," *Annals of Internal Medicine* 158, no. 4 (2013): 225–34.

16. Yan Zhang, Lu Lin, Huiling Li, Yan Hu, and Li Tian, "Effects of Acupuncture on Cancer-related Fatigue: A Meta-analysis," *Supportive Care in Cancer* 26, no. 2 (2017): 415–25.

17. Benjamin L. Hart and Lynette A. Hart, "How Mammals Stay Healthy in Nature: The Evolution of Behaviours to Avoid Parasites and Pathogens," *Philosophical Transactions of the Royal Society B: Biological Sciences* 373, no. 1751 (2018): 20,170,205.

18. Karl Shuker, *The Hidden Powers of Animals: Uncovering the Secrets of Nature* (Pleasantville, NY: Readers Digest, 2001).

19. Michael Greger and Gene Stone, *How Not to Die: Discover the Foods Scientifically Proven to Prevent and Reverse Disease* (New York: Flatiron Books, 2015).

20. Michael J. Hanley, Paul Cancalon, Wilbur W. Widmer, and David J. Greenblatt, "The Effect of Grapefruit Juice on Drug Disposition," *Expert Opinion on Drug Metabolism & Toxicology* 7, no. 3 (2011): 267–86.

21. Francesca Borrelli and Angelo A. Izzo, "Herb–Drug Interactions with St John's Wort (Hypericum Perforatum): An Update on Clinical Observations," *The AAPS Journal* 11, no. 4 (2009): 710–27.

22. Cecilia Amadi and Amaka A. Mgbahurike, "Selected Food/Herb-Drug Interactions: Mechanisms and Clinical Relevance," *American Journal of Therapeutics* 25, no. 4 (Jul/Aug 2018): e423–e433.

23. Borrelli and Izzo, "Herb–Drug Interactions with St John's Wort."

24. Ute Wölfle, Günter Seelinger, and Christoph Schempp, "Topical Application of St. John's Wort (Hypericum Perforatum)," *Planta Medica* 80, no. 02/03 (2013): 109–20.

25. Kevin C. Maki, Kerrie L. Kaspar, Christina Khoo, Linda H. Derrig, Arianne L. Schild, and Kalpana Gupta, "Consumption of a Cranberry Juice Beverage Lowered the Number of Clinical Urinary Tract Infection Episodes in Women with a Recent History of Urinary Tract Infection," *The American Journal of Clinical Nutrition* 103, no. 6 (2016): 1434–42.

26. Manisha Juthani-Mehta, Peter H. Van Ness, Luann Bianco, Andrea Rink, Sabina Rubeck, Sandra Ginter, Stephanie Argraves, Peter Charpentier, Denise Acampora, Mark Trentalange, Vincent Quagliarello, and Peter Peduzzi, "Effect of Cranberry Capsules

on Bacteriuria Plus Pyuria Among Older Women in Nursing Homes," *JAMA* 316, no. 18 (2016): 1879–87.

27. Jörg Melzer, Reto Brignoli, Curt Diehm, Jürgen Reichling, Dai-Do Do, and Reinhard Saller, "Treating Intermittent Claudication with Tibetan Medicine Padma 28: Does It Work?" *Atherosclerosis* 189, no. 1 (2006): 39–46.

28. Dan Bensky, Steven Clavey, and Erich Stöger, *Chinese Herbal Medicine* (Seattle, WA: Eastland Press, 2015).

## CHAPTER NINE: MY TREATMENT METHODS

1. Bryan Williams, Giuseppe Mancia, Wilko Spiering, Enrico Agabiti Rosei, Michel Azizi, Michel Burnier, Denis Clement, Antonio Coca, Giovanni De Simone, Anna Dominiczak, Thomas Kahan, Felix Mahfoud, Josep Redon, Luis Ruilope, Alberto Zanchetti, Mary Kerins, Sverre Kjeldsen, Reinhold Kreutz, Stephane Laurent, Gregory Y. H. Lip, Richard Mcmanus, Krzysztof Narkiewicz, Frank Ruschitzka, Roland Schmieder, Evgeny Shlyakhto, Konstantinos Tsioufis, Victor Aboyans, and Ileana Desormais, "2018 Practice Guidelines for the Management of Arterial Hypertension of the European Society of Cardiology and the European Society of Hypertension," *Journal of Hypertension* 36, no. 12 (2018): 2284–309.

2. W. A. Thomas, J. N. Davies, R. M. O'Neal, and A. A. Dimakulangan, "Incidence of Myocardial Infarction. A Geographic Study Based on Autopsies in Uganda, East Africa, and St. Louis, U.S.A.," *The American Journal of Cardiology* 5, no. 1 (February 1960): 41–47.

3. C. P. Donnison, "Blood Pressure in the African Native. Its Bearing upon the Aetiology of Hyperpiesia and Arterio-Sclerosis," *The Lancet* 213 (1929): 6–7.

4. Eric J. Topol and Steven E. Nissen, "Our Preoccupation with Coronary Luminology," *Circulation* 92, no. 8 (1995): 2333–42.

5. Dhanunjaya Lakkireddy, Donita Atkins, Jayasree Pillarisetti, Kay Ryschon, Sudharani Bommana, Jeanne Drisko, Subbareddy Vanga, and Buddhadeb Dawn, "Effect of Yoga on Arrhythmia Burden, Anxiety, Depression, and Quality of Life in Paroxysmal Atrial Fibrillation," *Journal of the American College of Cardiology* 61, no. 11 (2013): 1177–82.

6. Michael D. Sumner, Melanie Elliott-Eller, Gerdi Weidner, Jennifer J. Daubenmier, Mailine H. Chew, Ruth Marlin, Caren J. Raisin, and Dean Ornish, "Effects of Pomegranate Juice Consumption on Myocardial Perfusion in Patients With Coronary Heart Disease," *The American Journal of Cardiology* 96, no. 6 (2005): 810–14.

7. Tanjaniina Laukkanen, Hassan Khan, Francesco Zaccardi, and Jari A. Laukkanen, "Association Between Sauna Bathing and Fatal Cardiovascular and All-Cause Mortality Events," *JAMA Internal Medicine* 175, no. 4 (2015): 542–48.

8. Terence W. O'Neill, Paul S. McCabe, and John McBeth, "Update on the Epidemiology, Risk Factors and Disease Outcomes of Osteoarthritis," *Best Practice & Research Clinical Rheumatology* 32, no. 2 (2018): 312–26.

9. Romy Lauche, Nadine Gräf, Holger Cramer, Jallal Al-Abtah, Gustav Dobos, and Felix J. Saha, "Efficacy of Cabbage Leaf Wraps in the Treatment of Symptomatic Osteoarthritis of the Knee," *The Clinical Journal of Pain* 32, no. 11 (2016): 961–71.

10. A. H. Weinberger, M. Gbedemah, A. M. Martinez, D. Nash, S. Galea, and R. D. Goodwin, "Trends in Depression Prevalence in the USA from 2005 to 2015: Widening Disparities in Vulnerable Groups," *Psychological Medicine* 48, no. 08 (2017): 1308–15.

11. Ranja Stromberg, Estera Wernering, Anna Aberg-Wistedt, Anna-Karin Furhoff, Sven-Erik Johansson, and Lars G. Backlund, "Screening and Diagnosing Depression in Women Visiting GPs Drop in Clinic in Primary Health Care," *BMC Family Practice* 9, no. 1 (2008).

12. Peter C. Gøtzsche, *Deadly Psychiatry and Organised Denial* (København: People's Press, 2015).

13. Gøtzsche, *Deadly Psychiatry and Organised Denial*.

14. R. S. Opie, C. Itsiopoulos, N. Parletta, A. Sanchez-Villegas, T. N. Akbaraly, A. Ruusunen, and F. N. Jacka, "Dietary Recommendations for the Prevention of Depression," *Nutritional Neuroscience* 20, no. 3 (2016): 161–71.

15. Opie et al., "Dietary Recommendations for the Prevention of Depression," 161–71.

16. Ralph G. Walton, Robert Hudak, and Ruth J. Green-Waite, "Adverse Reactions to Aspartame: Double-blind Challenge in Patients from a Vulnerable Population," *Biological Psychiatry* 34, no. 1–2 (1993): 13–17.

17. Damian Hoy, Christopher Bain, Gail Williams, Lyn March, Peter Brooks, Fiona Blyth, Anthony Woolf, Theo Vos, and Rachelle Buchbinder, "A Systematic Review of the Global Prevalence of Low Back Pain," *Arthritis & Rheumatism* 64, no. 6 (2012): 2028–37.

18. Susanne Kaiser, "Themenseite: Rückenschmerzen," Statista Infografiken, accessed January 27, 2019, https://de.statista.com/themen/1364/rueckenschmerzen/.

19. Jan Hartvigsen, Mark Hancock, Alice Kongsted, Quinette Louw, Manuela Ferreira, Stephane Genevay, Damian Hoy, Jaro Karppinen, Glenn Pransky, Joachim Sieper, Rob Smeets, Martin Underwood, Rachelle Buchbinder, Dan Cherkin, Nadine E. Foster, Chris Maher, Maurits Tulder, Johannes R. Anema, Roger Chou, and Anthony Woolf, "What Low Back Pain Is and Why We Need to Pay Attention," *The Lancet* 391 (2018): 2356–67.

20. Hartvigsen et al., "What Low Back Pain Is," 2356–67.

21. Andrew J. Vickers, Emily A. Vertosick, George Lewith, Hugh Macpherson, Nadine E. Foster, Karen J. Sherman, Dominik Irnich, Claudia M. Witt, and Klaus Linde, "Acupuncture for Chronic Pain: Update of an Individual Patient Data Meta-Analysis," *The Journal of Pain* 19, no. 5 (2018): 455–74.

22. Christoph-Daniel Hohmann, Rainer Stange, Niko Steckhan, Sibylle Robens, Thomas Ostermann, Arion Paetow, and Andreas Michalsen, "The Effectiveness of Leech Therapy in Chronic Low Back Pain," *Deutsches Aerzteblatt International* 115, no. 47 (2018): 785–92.

23. "Worldwide Trends in Diabetes Since 1980: A Pooled Analysis of 751 Population-based Studies with 4.4 Million Participants," *The Lancet* 387, no. 10027 (2016): 1513–30.

24. "Worldwide Trends in Diabetes Since 1980," 1513–30.

25. "National Diabetes Statistics Report, 2017," Centers for Disease Control and Prevention, March 06, 2 018, accessed January 27, 2019, https://www.cdc.gov/diabetes/data/statistics-report/index.html.

26. Neal D. Barnard, Joshua Cohen, David Ja Jenkins, Gabrielle Turner-Mcgrievy, Lise Gloede, Amber Green, and Hope Ferdowsian, "A Low-fat Vegan Diet and a Conventional Diabetes Diet in the Treatment of Type 2 Diabetes: A Randomized, Controlled, 74-wk Clinical Trial," *The American Journal of Clinical Nutrition* 89, no. 5 (2009).

27. Hana Kahleova, Lenka Belinova, Hana Malinska, Olena Oliyarnyk, Jaroslava Trnovska, Vojtech Skop, Ludmila Kazdova, Monika Dezortova, Milan Hajek, Andrea Tura, Martin Hill, and Terezie Pelikanova, "Eating Two Larger Meals a Day (Breakfast and Lunch) Is More Effective than Six Smaller Meals in a Reduced-energy Regimen for Patients with Type 2 Diabetes: A Randomised Crossover Study," *Diabetologia* 57, no. 8 (2014): 1552–60.

28. Andreas Michalsen and Chenying Li, "Fasting Therapy for Treating and Preventing Disease—Current State of Evidence," *Forschende Komplementärmedizin / Research in Complementary Medicine* 20, no. 6 (2013): 444–53.

29. Lesya Marushka, Malek Batal, William David, Harold Schwartz, Amy Ing, Karen Fediuk, Donald Sharp, Andrew Black, Constantine Tikhonov, and Hing Man Chan, "Association Between Fish Consumption, Dietary Omega-3 Fatty Acids and Persistent Organic Pollutants Intake, and Type 2 Diabetes in 18 First Nations in Ontario, Canada," *Environmental Research* 156 (2017): 725–37.

30. H. Müller, F. Wilhelmi De Toledo, and K. L. Resch, "Fasting Followed by Vegetarian Diet in Patients with Rheumatoid Arthritis: A Systematic Review," *Scandinavian Journal of Rheumatology* 30, no. 1 (2001): 1–10.

31. Lucy Chen and Andreas Michalsen, "Management of Chronic Pain Using Complementary and Integrative Medicine," *BMJ* 357 (2017).

32. Augustine Amalraj, Karthik Varma, Joby Jacob, Chandradhara Divya, Ajaikumar B. Kunnumakkara, Sidney J. Stohs, and Sreeraj Gopi, "A Novel Highly Bioavailable Curcumin Formulation Improves Symptoms and Diagnostic Indicators in Rheumatoid Arthritis Patients: A Randomized, Double-Blind, Placebo-Controlled, Two-Dose, Three-Arm, and Parallel-Group Study," *Journal of Medicinal Food* 20, no. 10 (2017): 1022–30.

33. Chen and Michalsen, "Management of Chronic Pain Using Complementary and Integrative Medicine."

34. Daniel Furst, Manorama M. Venkatraman, Mary McGann, Ram Manohar, Cathryn Booth-LaForce, Reshmi Pushpan, P. G. Sekar, K. G. Raveendran, Anita Mahapatra, Jidesh Gopinath, and P. R. Krishna Kumar, "Double-Blind, Randomized, Controlled, Pilot Study Comparing Classic Ayurvedic Medicine, Methotrexate, and Their Combination in Rheumatoid Arthritis," *Journal of Clinical Rheumatology* 17, no. 4 (2011): 185–92.

35. Thomas De Rijdt, Isabel Spriet, Ludo Willems, Marianne Blanckaert, Martin Hiele, Alexander Wilmer, and Steven Simoens, "Appropriateness of Acid Suppression Therapy," *Annals of Pharmacotherapy* 51, no. 2 (2016): 125–34.

36. Amandeep Singh, Gail A. Cresci, and Donald F. Kirby, "Proton Pump Inhibitors: Risks and Rewards and Emerging Consequences to the Gut Microbiome," *Nutrition in Clinical Practice* 33, no. 5 (2018): 614–24.

37. Timothy P. Shiraev and Andrew Bullen, "Proton Pump Inhibitors and Cardiovascular Events: A Systematic Review," *Heart, Lung and Circulation* 27, no. 4 (2018): 443–50.

38. Avinash K. Nehra, Jeffrey A. Alexander, Conor G. Loftus, and Vandana Nehra, "Proton Pump Inhibitors: Review of Emerging Concerns," *Mayo Clinic Proceedings* 93, no. 2 (2018): 240–46.

39. Sara Pezeshkian and Susan E. Conway, "Proton Pump Inhibitor Use in Older Adults: Long-Term Risks and Steps for Deprescribing," *The Consultant Pharmacist* 33, no. 9 (2018): 497–503.

40. Timothy Card, Caroline Canavan, and Joe West, "The Epidemiology of Irritable Bowel Syndrome," *Clinical Epidemiology* 6 (2014): 71–80.

41. Shamsuddin M. Ishaque, S. M. Khosruzzaman, Dewan Saifuddin Ahmed, and Mukesh Prasad Sah, "A Randomized Placebo-controlled Clinical Trial of a Multi-strain Probiotic Formulation (Bio-Kult®) in the Management of Diarrhea-Predominant Irritable Bowel Syndrome," *BMC Gastroenterology* 18, no. 1 (2018): 71.

42. Susan A. Gaylord, Olafur S. Palsson, Eric L. Garland, Keturah R. Faurot, Rebecca S. Coble, J. Douglas Mann, William Frey, Karyn Leniek, and William E. Whitehead, "Mindfulness Training Reduces the Severity of Irritable Bowel Syndrome in Women:

Results of a Randomized Controlled Trial," *The American Journal of Gastroenterology* 106, no. 9 (2011): 1678–88.

43. Julie S. Phillips-Moore, Nicholas J. Talley, and Michael P. Jones, "The Mind-body Connection in Irritable Bowel Syndrome: A Randomised Controlled Trial of Hypnotherapy as a Treatment," *Health Psychology Open* 2, no. 1 (2015).


## CHAPTER TEN: STRATEGIES FOR A HEALTHY LIFE

1. Jacklyn K. Jackson, Amanda J. Patterson, Lesley K. Macdonald-Wicks, Christopher Oldmeadow, and Mark A. McEvoy, "The Role of Inorganic Nitrate and Nitrite in Cardiovascular Disease Risk Factors: A Systematic Review and Meta-analysis of Human Evidence," *Nutrition Reviews* 76, no. 5 (2018): 348–71.

2. "The Hispanic Paradox," *The Lancet* 385, no. 9981 (2015): 1918.

3. Mingyang Song, Teresa T. Fung, Frank B. Hu, Walter C. Willett, Valter D. Longo, Andrew T. Chan, and Edward L. Giovannucci, "Association of Animal and Plant Protein Intake With All-Cause and Cause-Specific Mortality," *JAMA Internal Medicine* 176, no. 10 (2016): 1453–63.

4. Michael Greger and Gene Stone, *How Not to Die: Discover the Foods Scientifically Proven to Prevent and Reverse Disease* (New York: Flatiron Books, 2015).

5. Nita G. Forouhi, "Consumption of Hot Spicy Foods and Mortality—Is Chilli Good for Your Health?" *BMJ* 351 (2015).

6. Magda Tsolaki, Elina Karathanasi, Ioulietta Lazarou, Kostas Dovas, Eleni Verykouki, Anastasios Karakostas, Kostas Georgiadis, Anthoula Tsolaki, Katerina Adam, Ioannis Kompatsiaris, and Zacharias Sinakos, "Efficacy and Safety of Crocus Sativus L. In Patients with Mild Cognitive Impairment: One Year Single-Blind Randomized, with Parallel Groups, Clinical Trial," *Journal of Alzheimers Disease* 54, no. 1 (2016): 129–33.


## CHAPTER ELEVEN: THE FUTURE OF MEDICINE

1. Nicholas J. Schork, "Personalized Medicine: Time for One-Person Trials," *Nature* 520, no. 7549 (2015): 609–11.

2. Trygve O. Tollefsbol, *Epigenetics in Human Disease* (London: Academic Press, 2012).

# Index

Page numbers in italics refer to illustrations and charts.

Hahn, Johann Siegmund, 51
Hahn, Siegmund, 51
Halle, Martin, 153
hawthorn, 235, 237, 244
hay fever, acupuncture treatment of, 228
hazelnuts, 273
headaches
　herbal medicines for, 237
　yoga and, 184
Head's zones, 226–27
healthy living, strategies for, 267–77
heart attacks
　bloodletting and, 41, 42
　exercise and, 152
　lessened sunlight exposure in northern
　　climates and, 5
　stress and, 174–75
heartburn, 235, 266
heat, 7–8
heat therapy. See hyperthermia
heavy metals, in Ayurvedic medicine, 222
heliotherapy. See sun bathing
hemochromatosis gene, 43
herbal medicine. See pharmacology and
　phytotherapy
Hesse, Hermann, 110
hibiscus tea, 242
high blood pressure (hypertension), 240–43
　author's treatment recommendations,
　　241–43
　bloodletting as treatment for, 41–42,
　　44–45, 242
　conventional medical treatment, 240–41
　exercise and, 242
　fasting and, 66, 88–89, 242
　hydrotherapy for, 57, 242–43
　meditation and, 242
　nature, beneficial health effects of
　　contact with, 156
　naturopathic treatment, 241
　olive oils and, 242
　superfoods/superdrinks for, 242
　vegetarian or vegan diet for, 241
　yoga and tai chi/qigong and, 184, 242
high fructose corn syrup, 127
Hildegard von Bingen, 204–5

Hildmann, Attila, 145
Hippocrates, 65, 115
hirudin, 29–30
homeodynamics, 16
homeopathy, xvi
honey, 11, 127, 275
hope, 21
hops, 236
hormesis
　cause and effect principle in research,
　　14–15
　cold and warm stimuli, reaction to, 7–12
　colds, treatment of, 1–2
　evolutionary connection between human
　　body and natural world, 7
　homeodynamics and, 12
　immune system balance, and seasonal
　　influences, 7
　living in harmony with nature, 6–8
　right stimulus at right intensity,
　　importance of, 2–3
　stress example, 15
　stress factors and protective reactions,
　　balance between, 7
　sunlight, exposure to, 4–6, 6
horseradish, 234, 237, 272
housekeeper effect, 80
humoral pathology, 27
hunger metabolism, 82
Hüther, Gerald, 81, 92, 95
hyaluronidase, 30
hydrotherapy, 49–59
　cardiac insufficiency (weak heart),
　　treatment of, 52–53
　colon hydrotherapies, 103
　compresses, 52, 58
　daily routine, integrating treatments
　　into, 57–59
　dew cure, 58–59
　high blood pressure, treatment of, 57
　historical use of, 50–51
　hypertension, treatment of, 242–43
　hypotension, treatment of, 57
　Kneipp's therapies, 8–9, 51–59
　mixture of warm and cold treatments, 54
　proper dosage, determining, 54–55

Kneipp therapies, 8–9, 51–59
  cardiovascular diseases and
    arteriosclerosis and, 246
  depression, treatment of, 251
*kōans*, 193
Kopf, Andreas, 22–23
Kräuchi, Kurt, 53–54
Kumar, Syal, 204, 211

lacto-vegetarian diet, 145
Langells, Otto, 182
lavender, 236
lavender extracts, 251–52
LDL cholesterol, 77, 147
lead, 87
leafy greens, 245, 253, 261, 271
lecithin, 132, 146
leech therapy, xviii, 25–37
  arthroses, treatment of, 33–35, 36, 37, 248
  back pain, treatment of, 36, 255–56
  bite of leeches, 28–29
  classification as drainage therapy, 26–27
  effectiveness of, 30–33
  hirudin, anti-coagulant and anti-
    inflammatory properties of, 29–30
  historical use of, 26–28
  osteoarthritis of knee, treatment of,
    31–33, 37
  patient case study (arthrosis), 33–35
  placebo effect of, 30
  procedures for applying leeches, 35–36
  secretions preventing harm to host, 29–30
  tennis elbow (epicondylitis), treatment
    of, 36
legumes, 145, 253, 259, 265, 274
Leitzmann, Claus, 122–23
Lemke, Harald, 149–50
lemon balm, 236
lemons, 136
lentils, 253, 259, 274
leptin, 88
lettuce, 271
Li, Qing, 155
Lichtenbelt, Wouter van Marken, 9–10
Liebig, Justus von, 120
Lifestyle Heart Trial, 116

"light" food products, 125
light therapy, 251
linden blossom tea, 2
lipolysis, 94
Liraglutide, 257
liver compresses, 103
liver disorders, herbal medicines for,
  235, 237
long-chain omega fatty acids, 119
Longo, Valter, 67–68, 70–72, 73, 93, 97, 105
lunch, 108
lung cancer, 16
Lustig, Robert, 126
lycopene, 253, 271
Lyon Diet Heart Study, 118–19
lysosome, 77

McClain, Donald A., 43
McGovern, George, 121
macronutrients, 120
Madeo, Frank, 78, 79, 80
*mala* (by-products and wastes), 209
manageability, 18
Mandela, Nelson, 19
Manohar, Ram, 217
mantras, 193, 200–201
Manz, Friedrich, 136–37
Mao Zedong, 205
massage cupping therapy, 40
massages
  connective tissue and, 160, 161, 162
  depression, treatment of, 252
Mattson, Mark, 86, 96, 104–5, 108
Mayr, Franz Xaver, 63, 144
Mayr's diet, 99–101
meals, timing of, 79–80
meaningfulness, 19
meat, 148–49
  acidic effect of, 136, 137
  amount consumed, 143
  animal fats, 121–22, 123
  classified as carcinogenic, 75
  from factory-farmed livestock, 123
  ferritin levels and, 43
  health risks related to consumption of,
    141–43

Salama, Abdulgabar, 44
Salonen, J. T., 44
salt, 7–8, 127–28
salutogenesis, 19, *20*
saturated fats, 77
saunas, 11, 53, 54–55
  cardiovascular diseases and
    arteriosclerosis and, 246
  *See also* hydrotherapy
sausages, 75, 128
Schedlowski, Manfred, 22
Schlenz, Maria, 11
Schlenz baths (hyperthermic baths), 11–12
Schork, Nicholas, 279
Schroth cure, 101
Schweninger, Ernst, 151–52
*Science,* 172
*Science of Fasting, The* (Gilman and
  Lestrade), 84
*The Science of Yoga: Risks and Rewards*
  (Broad), 186
Scotch hose therapy, 8, 9, 52, 55, *56,* 58.
  *See also* hydrotherapy
seeds, 121, 122
self-healing, 17–18
  deliberately inducing, 23–24
  fasting and, 86–87
  placebo effect and, 21–23
  sense of coherence and, 18–21
sense of coherence, 18–21
  comprehensibility criterion, 18
  doctor-patient relationship and, 19–21
  manageability criterion, 18
  meaningfulness criterion, 19
  salutogenesis theory and, 19, 20
serotonin, 81–82, 95, 253
Shaw, George Bernard, 61
*Shinrin-yoku* (forest bathing), 155, 251
Shirodhara therapy, 211–13
shivering, 8
short-chain omega fatty acids, 119
Shuhbeck, Alfons, 145
*Siddhartha* (Hesse), 110
siesta, 108
Singh, Rajinder, 198
sitting, 163

skin cancer, 4–5
sleep
  in cool rooms, 10
  digital screens and, 171
  herbal medicines for sleep disorders, 236
  stress and, 170–71
  warm feet and, 53–54, 58
smadhi, 189
snacking, 106–7
snow treading, 58–59
soft drinks, 124
Solomon, George, 180
sore throats, herbal medicines for, 234
soy, 121–22, 253
soybean oil, 118
soy oil, 245
spermidine, 79
spices, 10–11, 121, 209, 274–75. *See also*
  specific spices
spinach, 242, 271
spirituality, 19
spirituality, in Ayurvedic medicine, 221
St. John's wort, 233
stagnation, 16
Stapelfeldt, Elmar, 207, 217, 223
statins, 147
stem cells, 93
Steven, Sarah, 138
stimulus/dosage, 2–4
  cold and warm stimuli, 7–12
  patient's physical constitution and, 3–4
  right dosage, determining, 4–6
  stimulus-response principle (*See* hormesis)
  unspecific stimuli, 2–3
*Stone Age Is in Our Bones, The* (Ganten),
  72–73
strength training, 158–59
stress, 167–78
  body, effects on, *177*
  children and, 167
  constant availability and, 171–73
  diseases to which stress contributes, 175–76
  factors determining whether stress is
    healthy, 168
  fasting stress, 67, 92–93
  fear of, 174